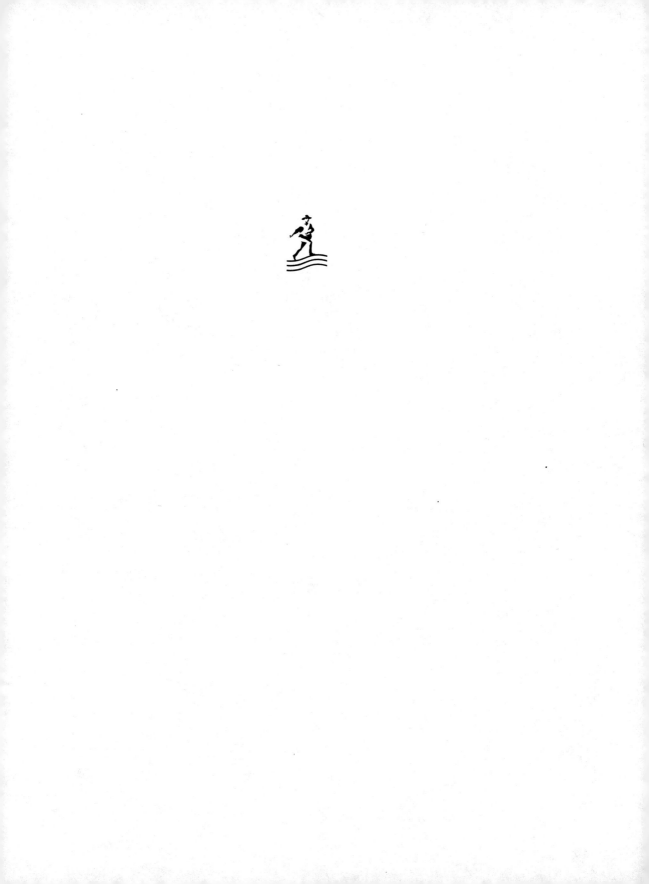

**Also by Terrell Owens**

*T.O.*

*Catch This!*

FOR CHILDREN

*Little T Learns to Share*

# T.O.'s FINDING FITNESS

*Making the Mind, Body, and
Spirit Connection for Total Health*

## Terrell Owens

with Buddy Primm and Courtney Parker

Foreword by Jerry Rice

Photography by Benjamin Fink

SIMON & SCHUSTER

New York   London   Toronto   Sydney

Simon & Schuster
1230 Avenue of the Americas
New York, NY 10020

First Simon & Schuster hardcover edition September 2008

SIMON & SCHUSTER and colophon are registered trademarks of Simon & Schuster, Inc.

For information about special discounts for bulk purchases, please contact Simon & Schuster Special Sales at 1-800-456-6798 or business@simonandschuster.com.

Childhood photographs (photo insert pages 1–4) are from the collection of the author's mother and are used with her permission. All other photographs are © Ben Fink.

*Designed by Joel Avirom and Jason Snyder*

Manufactured in the United States of America

10   9   8   7   6   5   4   3   2   1

Library of Congress Cataloging-in-Publication Data

Owens, Terrell, 1973–
  T.O's finding fitness : making the mind, body, and spirit connection for total health / Terrell Owens ; with Buddy Primm & Courtney Parker ; introduction by Jerry Rice.
    p. cm.
1. Physical fitness. 2. Nutrition. 3. Health. I. Primm, Buddy. II. Parker, Courtney. III. Title. IV. Title: Finding fitness.
  RA781.094 2008
  613.7'1—dc22   2008020742

ISBN-13: 978-1-4165-9512-0
ISBN-10:    1-4165-9512-0

*It's always funny to watch the reactions of people who ask me who my trainer is and I point to you. The thought that a stocky older, very southern white man is training me amazes them, and I laugh because I too am amazed. I know that I wouldn't be half the athlete I am today had it not been for you, Buddy. God put you in my life for a reason, and throughout the ten plus years we've been together, you've contributed most to my overall health and fitness regimen. You've taken me from an average athlete to one of the NFL's elite. Because of you and the information you've shared with me, I'm able to write this book. Thank you, Buddy, for making me better . . . mind, body, and spirit.*

# Acknowledgments

Getting in shape is never easy, but staying in shape can be even more challenging, which is why this book is so important. I've had so many instrumental people in my life who've assisted me in developing a fitness routine that not only worked but produced life-changing results.

First and foremost, I'd like to thank God, who truly is the source of my strength. Faith is key, and I have continued in the faith that allows my body to do extraordinary things.

I'd like to thank my family and friends, who keep me inspired to live my best life. I hope this book proves to be the first step at healthy and better lives for us all.

To my literary dream team: Joe Regal (you've proven to be the best so far), Michael Psaltis, Joe Carlone, Sydny Miner, and everyone at Simon & Schuster who made this process a smooth one, you've exceeded my expectations with this book. Many thanks.

To my football family: Jerry Jones and everyone at the Dallas Cowboys, thanks for making me a star! To my playmakers at Rosenhaus Sports, Drew, Jason, Robert . . . I consider you guys my dream team because you manage to make the impossible happen. They say it's not how you start but how you finish. Although I wish I had you all there from the start of my career, I'm grateful that our paths crossed when they did. Continue to give me your best because that's what you're gonna get from me.

Keith and everyone at the Estabrook Group: Image is everything! Thank you for helping me become just as good on the outside as I am on the inside.

The Hirsch family (thanks for letting us take over your house); Anthony Marotta of Luxury Rentals; Denine LeBat; John Lewis of Miami Beach Fitness; Ben Fink and Jeff Kavanaugh of Ben Fink Photography (so you *do* know the anatomy of the body); the management and staff of the Trump Palace Sunny Isles Beach, Florida; Rodrick Smith, Dennis and Louis Rodriguez, Barbara Becker, Liz Malm, Christopher and Victoria Murray (thanks for all your help); Kari Pinnock, and everyone else that helped us out in Miami during the Finding Fitness photo shoot, thank you.

Blake Kassel of Bodylastics, thanks for helping me create such an excellent product. The T.O. Super Strong Man Bands are truly amazing!

To Courtney Parker: I really don't know where to begin, but I guess that's the beauty of our fifteen-year friendship. Our careers have taken us to heights unimaginable. We've watched each other grow, and along the way we've done it all by the grace of God and our faith in Him and each other. Who would have thought that in all this time of finding fitness, I would also find a friend in you. You are the best!

Finally, to everyone who either has or will contribute to my overall fitness . . . without you this wouldn't be a reality. Thank you for helping me always find fitness and be fit for life.

## Buddy's Acknowledgments

First of all, I want to thank God. None of this would be possible without His blessings.

Of course, I want to thank Terrell. You've been like a son to me. It's been both an honor and pleasure working with you to achieve your professional goals. Thank you for your dedicated training and commitment to fitness and me, which provided the basis for this book. This is a dream come true. Thank you for this wonderful opportunity.

To Courtney Parker, thank you for your unwavering dedication to the cause as well as your patience with all of us throughout this entire process. You are an extraordinary talent, and without you this wouldn't be possible.

Behind every good man is a good woman, and my wife, Mary, is just that for me. Thank you for always supporting everything I do.

Thanks to Blake and Victoria for all your help.

Last but not least, I want to thank each and every one of my clients over the past thirty years. You all keep me inspired to live my best life.

## Courtney's Acknowledgments

So many people were instrumental in making this book possible. I'd say ditto to everyone Terrell and Buddy already acknowledged. I've learned so much from this experience that has assisted me in making my own mind, body, and spirit connection. This is an awesome book. I thank God for always increasing my blessings in every area so that I may be a blessing to others. Thank you all so much!

To Terrell: Well, I guess we can check off another item from our list of things to do. (LOL) I am honored to call you my friend. Thanks for always challenging me to be better, believing in me when I'm in doubt, and encouraging me to stay strong in the face of adversity. I know that I am a better woman because of you.

# Contents

# Foreword

JERRY RICE

In 1985, as a first-round pick by the San Francisco 49ers in the NFL draft, I boarded a plane for the first time in my life and began to practice with the greatest team ever assembled. Having been drafted high from a small southern school, Mississippi Valley State, I had something to prove. The team, under the direction of head coach Bill Walsh and then George Seifert, developed a winning formula for how to practice, how to play, and how to act. As part of that process, the veterans passed on their knowledge of football and of "the 49er way" to the rookies. I was in awe of Joe Montana, Roger Craig, and Dwight Clark, and I soaked up everything I could. When I struggled mightily out of the gate, the veterans and Bill Walsh picked me up.

By 1996, the 49ers had already won three Super Bowls on the shoulders of giants like Montana, Craig, Clark, Steve Young, and Ronnie Lott. Given my own experience, when another high-draft-pick wide receiver from a small southern school joined the 49ers in 1996, I took a keen interest. Terrell Owens played at the University of Tennessee at Chattanooga, not exactly a football power similar to Mississippi Valley State. (I didn't know it at the time, but Terrell had chosen to wear number 80 — my number — in honor of his favorite receiver.) The young man from Alexandria, Alabama, had had a difficult childhood, yet managed to excel in any and all sports. Football was a passion, and, as he developed at UTC, the NFL scouts took notice. He put up decent-but-not-great numbers his senior year, mostly due to double teams by opponents, but the 49ers took a chance — again — on a good-sized wide receiver from a small school.

It might come as a bit of surprise to those of you who now know Terrell as T.O., but he was a quiet, shy kid when he arrived at the 49er camp, in awe of his new teammates, as I had been more than ten years earlier. He had a chance to listen and learn during that first season with the Niners; he watched the receivers break in stride, he watched as we finished every play in practice and games, he watched as we treated the game as our job. One of the first things I noticed about Terrell was his work ethic. He was always picking my brain about how to run a route better or how to extend his fingers when making a catch. He busted his butt in practice and in the weight room. At 6 foot 3 and 200-plus pounds, Terrell wanted to add muscle to be more effective off the line of scrimmage against defensive backs, so every day, before or after practice, you could find him in the weight room, benching, squatting, and doing just about everything else imaginable with a free weight. Despite his willingness to learn and work hard at the wide receiver position, Terrell saw action mainly on special teams in the first months of that first season. He felt he had something to prove, and he excelled, even had three special-team tackles in a game against Atlanta.

When one of our receivers, J. J. Stokes, went down with an injury in October 1996, Terrell stepped up and, in his first game against Cincinnati, hauled in four catches for 94 yards, including a 45-yard touchdown. He never looked back. As the seasons progressed, Terrell became stronger, faster, and a more precise receiver, and his numbers exploded. My career with San Francisco wound down, and I remember my final home game against the Chicago Bears in December 2000. The 49er fans were so gracious to me that day, but it was Terrell who was the star. He caught *twenty* passes for 283 yards. After the game, when the team awarded me the game ball on my special day, I, in turn, passed the ball on to Terrell. It was his team now.

Despite his stardom, Terrell has never turned his back on what helped get him to the top: hard work. He still hits the gym and the track on the hot summer days as he did as a rookie in 1996. He knew early on that fitness was not only key to being a better player but essential for a more durable and longer-lasting career.

When I played for San Francisco, my off-season workouts on the hills of California became legendary. Though I no longer play football, every day that my schedule permits, I am in the gym by 7:30 A.M. Three times a week, I do two hours of cardio—bike, stairs, treadmill; the other days I hit the weights. Like Terrell, I understand the importance of taking care of your body and mind, eating right, having an exercise regimen, and putting a positive spin on your day. I keep myself in shape not only because it helps prevent injuries but because I know that it takes a lot more work to get back into shape than it does to stay in shape!

Fitness is focus. When I am at the gym, you won't see me listening to an iPod or watching *SportsCenter* on TV, unlike almost every other gym patron I see. I don't need the distractions. I am so focused on my workout and what I need to accomplish that time flies by. Focus leads to a better workout, which in turn leads to better fitness.

Staying fit is a *lifestyle* choice. It is more than a daily trip to the gym. It's about taking the stairs instead of the elevator; ordering water instead of soda; asking yourself, "Is this good for my body?" before making a choice. I've made the lifestyle choice, and so has Terrell.

Beyond the hype, the touchdown celebrations, and the flash, Terrell is the same young man I met in 1996, with the drive, passion, and commitment necessary for excellence. He has become one of the best wide receivers of all time, and he will continue to make his mark in the record books. A core reason for his success, even after twelve years in the game, is that Terrell knows, and understands, the importance of fitness.

Now, if I can only get that 2000 game ball back from T.O.!

# T.O.'s
# FINDING
# FITNESS

# Introduction

It all starts with the mind.

Have you ever wondered how a young child can do a back flip without anyone teaching him? If a five-year-old sees an older kid do a back flip and makes up his mind that he wants to do it too, that child is often able to mimic what he just saw. The eyes send a message to the brain, the brain instructs the body, and by instinct the body responds to what the mind tells it to do.

For years people have asked me what method I used to get into such incredible shape, and my answer has always been simple: Think about what you really want to accomplish. Tell your body what you want it to do, and then do it!

That may sound simplistic, but it really isn't. Physical success starts with the mind. It's a remarkably straightforward and effective approach that anyone can use. For instance, I didn't always have this body; as a teen I was tall and lanky. Even in my early days in the NFL, my body was a little above average at best. Yet no matter what I lacked in size, mentally I knew my body could do extraordinary things. That mental focus—not natural physical prowess—is how I went from an undeveloped rookie to the NFL's number one wide receiver. And it's what I'm going to teach you in this book.

*Finding Fitness* will show you how to use the power of your mind to lose weight and get into your best shape. But more than that, this book will help you love *your* body and unlock the door to your untapped abilities. *Finding Fitness* is the tool that will help you unleash the You you were designed to be.

Whether you're a stay-at-home mom, a college student, a weekend athlete, or an NFL star, *Finding Fitness* will help you make the mind-body connection that will ultimately bring out your own best body.

## MIND OVER MATTER—SHOW VERSUS TELL

I could easily write a book that simply tells you about my workout, my lifestyle, and my diet. But that wouldn't be the best way to help you.

My approach emphasizes more show than tell. The mind understands one thing: Either I can do what I see, or I cannot. For me, "cannot" is not an option. I'm going to show you how to determine the most effective way for *you* to get into shape, rather than just tell you what works for me. Once you learn how to make your own success instead of just reading about how I became successful, you'll be on your way to discovering the fitness routine and eating plan that works best for you.

My hope is to get you to move past the superficial expectations set by others, and determine and achieve goals that will make you happy.

I've found that for me, the best method of learning is sight recognition, then verbal or written instruction, and then trial and (sometimes) error, repetition, and ultimately perfection. That is the method I will employ in this book.

With each exercise, I'm going to first provide a visual example of form at a beginner level, an intermediate level, and an advanced level. Each photograph focuses on an important aspect of the exercise so you can see exactly what's happening during each movement.

My personal trainer and fitness expert, Buddy Primm, offers tips and techniques for getting the most out of each exercise.

Buddy also provides easy-to-follow diet and exercise plans based on his many years of personal training, as well as my twelve years in the NFL working extensively with NFL trainers and doctors. Some people search their entire lives to find the knowledge about fitness that is provided in the pages of this book!

I'll share some of my best moments and some of my worst, including accounts and illustrations of some very serious career-threatening injuries. I will show and tell you how I overcame those injuries and persevered through those challenging times.

## HOW I'LL CHANGE THE WAY YOU THINK ABOUT FITNESS

I believe fitness is individual: It should never be patterned after someone else's body or lifestyle. You can't just look at me and say, "I want Terrell's body." What you should say is "I want *my* body to look that fit and healthy, and I can do what he does in order to get there." *That's* achievable!

With my help, you'll be able to determine what balance of exercises gives you the results *you* want instead of what someone else's program says you should achieve. You'll also begin to ask yourself questions about food—what can it do for and to your body—as well as understand why your body responds to food in certain ways. This book will give you the mental capabilities to accomplish your physical goals.

*Finding Fitness* can work for you whether you want to lose ten pounds or two hundred. Beyond weight loss, it can help you change behaviors that are not working. If you can find the things in life that make you happy and can push through and past the things that cause you distress, you will achieve the extraordinary success that all of us were intended to have. Now let's get started!

# PART I

## Making the Mind, Body, Spirit Connection

**1**

---

# The Mind! Understanding
# the Mind-Body Connection

**When I first entered the NFL,** I never imagined that being a professional athlete would be my life. I grew up poor in a small southern town in Alabama and honestly never gave much thought to who I'd become.

I always knew I'd do something, but I never planned out what that would be.

As fate would have it, the body that I hated as a teen has become one of my greatest assets in life. But it didn't start there, it started with my mind.

Your mind controls your thoughts and your emotions, which ultimately control your actions. If you indulge in negative thoughts and emotions, the end result will be that your actions are negative too.

If you plant the mental seed of a healthy body—no matter what shape you're in now—it will eventually manifest. So before we get started on your body, let's first make you "thought strong" so that you can be strong in your mind, then we can make you strong in your body.

I've found that the easiest way to enhance your strengths is to first be able to identify your weaknesses. So many times people focus on what they want without committing to what it's going to take to achieve that goal. I've become the athlete that I am today by taking the focus off what I feel are my greatest assets and instead have turned my attention to the areas where I need to change the most. Since this book is about finding fitness, it is important to review the factors that are stopping you from achieving your fitness goals.

On the following pages is a list of seven challenges that will keep you from fulfilling your goals of optimum health and fitness. Identify what is holding you back; then study, tackle, and conquer each one, once and for all.

**1. Fear:** *to feel fear in oneself, to have an unpleasant, often strong emotion caused by anticipation or awareness of something uncertain; to be afraid or apprehensive.*

Fear is the number one cause of an unhealthy lifestyle. Fear monopolizes your thoughts and immobilizes your ability to achieve your goals.

Fear is a learned behavior and not a natural instinct.

I often use the analogy of a child daring to do something that he or she has never done before, because most children, especially at a young age, haven't yet learned to incorporate fear into their equation of life. Part of my success came from not fearing what I wanted to accomplish. Instead of saying "Oh, woe is me!" I adopted the mind-set of "why *not* me?" If Jerry Rice and Michael Jordan could be two of the best athletes in their sports, so could I. Period.

Where there is fear, it is impossible to focus. Ask yourself what you're afraid of as it relates to fitness, and reverse your thinking about whatever that is to achieve your goals. You can do anything you set your mind to. How you think reflects who you are, so think only the best.

**2. Doubt:** *uncertainty of belief or opinion that often interferes with decision making; a deliberate suspension of judgment.*

It is my belief that fear and doubt are related. In order to achieve total health, you have to believe you can find a fitness regimen that works for you. I can always tell when I'm working with a champion who is serious about changing as opposed to someone who will probably never get further than just talking about change; a champion believes the words he or she is saying and puts them into action.

I remember coaches telling me in my rookie year, "If you do this and work out this way, you'll be a star."

I accepted those words; I wanted to be the best, and I never doubted that I would be. There are going to be times in your life when something may seem challenging, even downright difficult, but never allow the level of challenge to make you doubt it can be done.

If you're looking to lose weight—no matter how many pounds you're talking about—you have to trust yourself. Don't focus on the "how to" part. Wrap your mind around the "can do" part first. Once you believe that you can lose weight, the "how to" part will come more easily.

**3. Rejection:** *the act or process of rejecting; the state of being rejected; something or someone being left out or denied.*

Anything from a failed relationship to not getting picked for a team—even the denial of credit—can affect you physically. Rejection of any sort can lead you to an unhealthy place of depression or negativity. That state is usually followed by the absence of physical activity and a disordered diet.

Moving on from rejection to complete fitness fulfillment isn't as difficult as you may think. It does, however take effort to develop the determination that you will never allow one *no* to spoil an entire lifetime of potential *yesses*.

**4. Delay:** *the act of delaying; inactivity resulting in something being put off until a later time.*

I love the definition of this word. Step 4 is probably the most popular explanation never given. You heard me right, never given. The reason I say this is because the person who uses it probably hasn't gotten around to giving it.

As a child I lived by the saying "Never put off until tomorrow what you can do today." The reason I love this advice so much is that it's true. Time is the most valuable asset any human being has. To mentally prepare to find your level of true fitness, you have to adopt a mind-set that doesn't allow you to waste time on making the decision to be fit. Once you decide to get in the game, you can play! But you have to make the decision to do it.

**5. Ignorance:** *the lack of knowledge or education*

I'm amazed that so many people don't exercise or have a healthy diet because they lack the understanding of what it truly means to stay in shape. You have to know yourself. For example, if a person is challenged with an illness or injury, they may come up with their own solution to the problem or try to self-medicate, rather than seek professional advice concerning their condition. When a friend of mine was challenged with a hamstring injury, instead of seeking professional help and treating the injury accordingly with the proper rehabilitation and special care, he relied only on his own knowledge, which not only delayed healing but at one point actually worsened his condition.

It is important to read and study everything you can about health and exercise before it becomes an issue for you, rather than when your weight and health become a problem and you're desperate for results.

Don't be one of those people who waits until a doctor says, "If you don't start eating better, you're going to die!" Learn and apply the necessary steps before that time so that you are always safe and never sorry.

**6. Time:** *the continuum of experience in which events pass from the future through the present to the past.*

I'll keep this simple: people make time for what they want to make time for. If you can make time to watch one thirty-minute sitcom or an hour-long drama on TV, you can find at least twenty minutes a day to take care of your body. The reality is that you get only one body, so find the time to do right by it.

**7. Excuse:** *a poor example; a defense of some offensive behavior or some failure to keep a promise.*

The number one excuse for not working out is *any* excuse for not working out.

In order to build a solid foundation and establish a lifestyle of fitness, you have to focus on finding a fitness routine that will work for you. To do this, you have to tackle the weaknesses that keep you from moving forward.

My suggestion? Identify each issue, write it down, and then, for ten days, work on the obstacle that stands in your way. Tackle that mental mountain head-on, and verbally assault anything that's hindering your growth with a positive affirmation of hope. Where there is hope, there is also healing. Step by step, you can and will overcome the mental challenges that keep you from reaching and maintaining you fitness goals. Take the first step today!

## T.O. TESTIMONY: *Truly a Rookie*

When I first stepped into the locker room of the 49ers, I was in complete awe. I couldn't believe I was there and that my locker was directly next to that of a man I'd admired for so long, Jerry Rice. To think that my idol would now become my mentor was more than I could stand. But there I stood, ready to face the challenge, willing to do the work, and anxious for an opportunity to play.

During my rookie year I was shy, quiet, and humble. I didn't walk in like I had something to prove (even though I did); I walked into training camp as if I had everything to learn. I knew early on that if I wanted to become even a fraction of the man who stood next to me, I had to be quick to listen and slow to speak. I laugh when I hear reports about the difference between Terrell Owens (the rookie) and T.O. (the seasoned vet). People say that I've changed, but change is always inevitable. What most people don't know is that when you change how you think about a thing, you also change how you are. The only confidence I had coming into the league was that obviously I was meant to be there. If I was going to succeed, I would have to dig deep and develop my body to function as a star.

When you're in the growing-up phase of life, it's important to listen and learn everything you can about what you're going to do. As a rookie, I had nothing to say but everything to do.

I took advice from people like Jerry Rice and Bill Walsh and respected my team. I waited for my chance on the field, and even though my position was wide receiver, most of my playing time early on was on special teams.

I remember that in the game against Atlanta, I had three tackles and thought to myself, "I'm supposed to be on offense, not on defense." Every game I played—before, during and after, no matter the outcome—I'd say to myself, "If I keep working hard, my opportunity will come." If I didn't play my position or have much game time, I trained harder. When team practice was over, for me it had just begun. I stayed late, worked out. I prayed a lot, knowing my chance would come. It did!

My teammate J. J. Stokes, number 83, got injured, and I was set to start in the game against Cincinnati. Most of the game was a blur: play after play, snap after snap, run after run; I was in position. Four passes, 94 yards, and a 45-yard touchdown play to tie the game. I was no longer just a rookie. The game, for me, had changed.

---

# The Body! Knowing What
# Your Body Can Do

**A girl jokingly asked me the other day** if I ever look at myself in the mirror and wonder, "Do I look fat?" I laughed and told her no. What I realize about my body now is that instead of working harder I have to work smarter in order to achieve the best results. I do, however, look at myself with the wisdom I have about my body today and think, "If only I'd known then what I know now." I would've been deadly as a rookie with the understanding I have now of how my body functions.

One of the main aims of this book is to help *you* get a better understanding of yourself so that you can push to the next level. Having worked with some of the greatest doctors, trainers, and nutritional experts in the world, I want everyone reading this book to understand the practical knowledge that has helped me transform my natural body into an amazing machine and learn to apply it in their own lives.

It won't cost you hundreds of thousands of dollars to achieve your goals. The only price you have to pay is what it will cost you in time and effort.

When you go to the doctor, who does he or she consult with to determine what's wrong with you? You. You're the only expert on your body. You know what you can and cannot do, based on what you've decided you want to do.

When I'm asked to run a play and learn a route, in the back of my mind I understand that there are several opposing factors (and people) trying to stand in the way of my accomplishing that goal. Yet no matter what—or who—is trying to move against me, I've already made up my mind that I can run the play successfully. I'm prepared for the defense's strategy, and my body is ready and willing to go all the way with me. I've set my mind to achieve my goal.

It's important to know that your body, if you allow it to be, is on your side. It has the power to work with you and doesn't have to work against you. If you take the time to study and listen to your body and what it needs to survive and be strong, you'll discover exactly what your body can do.

*Too often* I see young athletes giving 100 percent to exercise. Yet by consuming fast foods on a daily basis, they are negating their efforts by not considering the importance of a healthy diet.

The excuse I often hear from these young people is, "It costs too much to eat healthy, and I need to eat as much as possible in order to put on the size I need for my position."

There are two things wrong with that statement. First, eating healthy is probably the *least* expensive thing anyone can ever do. However, it's the most valuable thing you will ever do. Second, the more junk food you consume, the harder it is to break the habit later in life, when your body doesn't need all the extra calories.

I'll save most of this for the diet and menu section, but I do want to point out two things.

The money you end up spending when you eat out or buy and cook foods high in fat is no less than what you spend on food that is better for you. Example: An average person at a local fast-food restaurant will spend approximately $5.00 to $10.00 on a single meal. For most college athletes, that's nothing but a snack, even if you're cruising the $1.00 menu.

Let's do the math:

$1.00 burger / sandwich x 2 + $1.00 fries + $1.00 drink + $1.00 dessert = $5.00 — and that's for *one* snack or meal!

Now buy a $2.00 bag of apples (usually four to six apples) + a $1.00 loaf of bread, + $2.00 for about four cans of tuna + $1.00 for a large bag of baked potato chips + $0.00 for a glass of water = $6.00 — for approximately three to four snacks or meals. You get the point. I want to stop the misconception once and for all that eating healthy is expensive. That is not true.

The body is our most important tool; we control what goes into it and what comes out.

I usually don't offer much of an opinion about alcohol and drugs, but I will go on the record now and say this: every decision you make regarding your body has consequences that affect you and everyone around you. I make choices that will allow my body to perform at a maximum capacity, using only natural substances. I don't want to upset my body's ability to function naturally, so I'm extremely careful about what I consume.

We only get one body in this lifetime, and I encourage you to do what is right by yours now. It's never too late to make a midcourse correction in regard to the health of your body. Strength is an asset that radiates both inside and out. The following affirmations will help you remember just how strong you truly are.

### Strength Affirmations for Your Body

1. I have a champion's body.

2. I eat what is right.

3. I know that I am a winner.

4. My body is healthy and strong.

5. I make wise choices regarding food.

6. I am a whole, healthy_____ pounds.

7. My body functions the way it is supposed to function.

8. I have complete confidence in my body.

9. I can overcome any physical challenge.

To some this may seem corny, but affirming those things is a great way to achieve confidence in your body and set a standard of wholeness for yourself every day of your life.

**T.O. TESTIMONY:** *The First Injury*

It was the 1999 wild-card play-off round, and the 49ers were hosting the Green Bay Packers. Steve Young was trying not to lose his mind after I had dropped the ball several times. The way I was catching—or rather not catching—was about to hand Green Bay the victory.

With less than two minutes to play in the game and the 49ers down by four, Steve did everything he could to keep us alive, which meant not throwing the ball to me.

On a third-down-and-three play at the Packers' 25, Steve stumbled yet threw a bullet into the end zone for a 49ers touchdown with three seconds remaining on the clock.

The receiver on the play was me! I caught that ball even though I'd been hit by two Packers defenders. I crashed into the ground, and that play resulted in the first of many high ankle sprains. The severity of pain was nothing compared to the joy I felt in knowing that I'd actually caught that ball—a catch that would ultimately advance us to the play-offs and change my position and place in the NFL forever.

I knew then that no matter what injury came against me during a game, God's graces and proper training would determine who I'd become as a player and just what my body could do. I remember that pain as if it were yesterday. The throbbing, the swelling, the agony. But despite the pain, the only thing running through my mind was that I'd just caught the ball and I still had it in my hand. My catch had just won us the game.

Fitness starts with the mind, and then the body responds. My body responded to the joy of my victory because that was my focus instead of the pain in my ankle. From the first injury to (hopefully) the last, as long as you can believe that healing starts first in the mind, victory in any circumstance is possible.

## THE 10 MOST COMMON FOOTBALL INJURIES

I've played sports since I was five. All that mattered to me was running, jumping, hitting, crashing into something or someone: if an activity had all that, I was in.

After years in the league watching fellow players and personally experiencing the breaks and bruises the NFL has to offer, I thought I'd share some of the most common injuries in football with the hope of shedding some light on the choices I've made as they relate to my career and giving you some insight into why it's necessary to be prepared mentally and physically for all that life has to offer.

## A DAY IN THE LIFE OF A TRUE BALLER

The reason that there are so many rules governing football is that the potential for injury is so great. Tackles and falls can lead to sprains, breaks, and concussions. Broken noses are also a common problem, despite the fact that we should and are required to wear protective gear. Other injuries include but are not limited to

- Neck injuries
- Tendonitis
- Sprains and breaks
- Shoulder injuries/dislocations
- Hand injuries/broken or torn ligaments
- Cervical spine injuries
- Knee injuries
- Clavicle fractures
- Muscle pulls
- ACL tears

No matter how invincible you think you are, there is absolutely no escaping injuries while you are seriously working out or playing professional sports. Below are photos of some of my real-life injuries, along with tips and exercises that I used to rehab and strengthen my body to experience a full recovery.

## INJURY 1. MEDICAL TERM: CLAVICLE FRACTURE

**Layman's term:** Broken collarbone

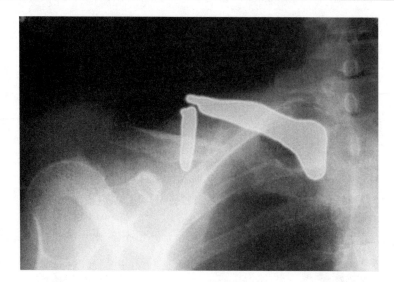

**ESTIMATED RECOVERY TIME:** Season-ending

**ACTUAL RECOVERY TIME:** 8 weeks

**WHAT WE DID:** We placed a pin into my lateral clavicle fragment with a drill. Under X-ray control the drill was attached to the exiting end and redirected to pin the full length of the clavicle. Finally, a screw and washer were put into the fracture to hold the bone in place.

**IMPACT ON CAREER:** Became an Eagle, career soared.

**WHAT HAPPENED NEXT:** Moved to Dallas, became a star!

### "IT'S OVER FOR OWENS!"
DECEMBER 23, 2003

Wide receiver Terrell Owens broke his left collarbone against Philadelphia on Dec. 21. Owens was injured after catching a 20-yard pass and getting tackled by safety Brian Dawkins. He immediately went to the locker room, where X-rays revealed the injury. Barring some terrible misjudgment, this injury could signal the end of his career as a 49er.

## INJURY 2. MEDICAL TERM: DELTOID LIGAMENT SPRAIN AND MAISONNEUVE FRACTURE

**Layman's term:** Ankle/leg injury

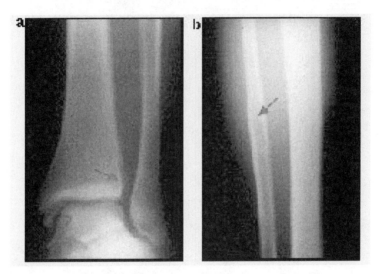

**ESTIMATED RECOVERY TIME:** 10–12 weeks

**ACTUAL RECOVERY TIME:** 6 weeks

**WHAT WE DID:** We inserted two screws into my right ankle and a plate on the outside of the ankle.

**FEELING AFTER I PLAYED IN MY FIRST SUPER BOWL GAME:** Indescribable.

**WORTH IT:** Absolutely.

### "TO PLAY OR NOT TO PLAY"
#### DECEMBER 20, 2004

Owens was hurt on the second play of the third quarter in the Eagles' win over the Dallas Cowboys when he was dragged down from behind by Roy Williams. During the 20-yard reception, Owens' leg was dislocated. Although Owens plans to be in uniform for the big game, the ultimate decision on T.O.'s status will be left up to the doctors and training staff.

## INJURY 3. MEDICAL TERM: METACARPAL FRACTURE

**Layman's term:** Broken finger

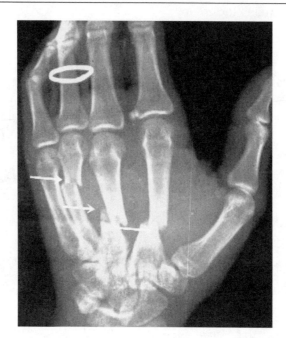

**ESTIMATED RECOVERY TIME:** 4–6 weeks

**ACTUAL RECOVERY TIME:** 10 days

**WHAT WE DID:** A metal plate and screws were inserted to stabilize the fourth metacarpal of my right hand. They were left in the hand even after the break healed, not to be taken out unless they caused irritation or infection, or if excess scar tissue needed to be removed.

**READY FOR GAME DAY:** You better believe it.

**CATCHPHRASE AFTER THE GAME:** Getcha popcorn ready!

**"OWENS BREAKS FINGER, OUT FOUR TO SIX WEEKS"**

SEPTEMBER 18, 2006

Owens flubbed a pass in the end zone on the opening drive and by game's end, he was in the locker room getting his hand X-rayed, his stats sealed at three catches for 19 yards. The X-rays revealed the break.

# 3

# The Spirit! The Source of My Strength

**It is no secret that I have a bit of a reputation.** It's comical, because in some of my most controversial moments, it's been my faith that has protected me from my sometimes worst enemy: myself.

I'm reminded of every time I missed the mark—in my relationships with my family, my friends, and even my teams—and had to use my faith to make my crooked path straight. People often ask me, "How do you keep going? How do you overcome the adversity that seems to await you at every corner?"

My answer is simple: Faith is the key!

When I was young, my grandmother never allowed me many luxuries. I learned the hard lessons of lack very early on. An appreciation of the little things was a trait I adopted quickly, and to this day I love both my mother's and grandmother's sternness, for it made me who I am. When there was nothing else to do—or rather nothing more I *could* do—I would read the Bible and pray for a better situation.

This chapter isn't here to promote religion; it's simply to urge you to get in touch with *your* spirit and what you can achieve.

One of my favorite passages in scripture states that one should always watch and pray in order not to fall into temptation, for the spirit is willing but the flesh is weak.

I look back over my life and think about the times when my own flesh was weak, and this verse gives me strength. We've all been there. Personally, I've had moments when I've been weak with uncertainty, weak as a result of my poor choices, weak with failures, even weak with extreme injuries, and through it all my spirit has sustained me.

To truly find fitness, you have to tap deep within yourself to discover faith. Faith will ultimately get you to a place of empowerment. God is and always has been my source of strength. My spirit and faith have allowed me to experience awesome things.

The stronger you are in body, the stronger you'll become in spirit. Your spirit comes alive when your body has the energy to shoulder the pressures of this world. Through the pages of this book, my desire is to help you make the connection between your mind and body. Once you do that, you'll understand that your spirit is the final link to an unbreakable chain that is the new you.

# PART II

## Show Versus Tell

**4**

# What It All Means

I hope the previous chapters have helped prepare you for what's to come. It's important to embrace the mind-body-spirit connection. Everything starts with the mind. Everything! If you set your mind on high things, you'll achieve high goals. Of course, the opposite is true as well. Lack of ambition and negative thoughts will deliver negative results in every area of your life.

Once you overcome your mental weaknesses, affirm that your body can do remarkable things, and tap into the spirit within yourself, you will be one step closer to making a complete transformation that will lead you to a lifestyle of fitness forever.

## GAME TIME

### Steps to Finding Fitness

1. Identify which mental challenges have been holding you back from discovering your true path to fitness.

2. Write them down and use them as your mental playbook for conquering your fitness goals.

3. Spend ten days before you begin a new program mentally preparing yourself for your workout.

4. Make the decision that no matter where you start, you will make the commitment to stay with your program for at least two weeks straight.

5. Allow your body to dictate your progress. Do not focus on what others are doing. Stay the course, maintain your own flow. This is about *your* lifestyle, and it will take time to create.

6. Lose the rules. Fitness shouldn't be about rules; it should be about using your natural tools (mind, body, and spirit) to create the energy and space in which you want to live. When you can truly say you're comfortable in your own skin and with yourself, you have succeeded in finding fitness.

7. Create an atmosphere of confidence. Take time to really get to know what you like and dislike about working out. Some people enjoy working out at the gym. Others prefer to stay home and work out alone. For some, a one-on-one program with a trainer may be best. There is no right or wrong; you can and will get results lifting weights, doing pilates at home, or using my personal gym system. What you do and where you do it is determined by your schedule, your current lifestyle, your strengths and weaknesses, and your goals.

It's more important that you change your mind and your thinking about what it takes to be fit than to focus on the hows, whys, whens, and wheres of how you're going to do it. Making the decision to live a lifestyle geared to fitness is the most important step you will take toward achieving your goals.

Now that you're mentally strong, let's get down to what's real. No matter where you start or stop, you're already a winner.

One final thought: I want you to understand that the reason my body can withstand the damage that can be done in the NFL, and the reason I've managed to come back from what other people would consider career-ending injuries, is that I believe in focusing on strengthening and developing the core—that is, working muscles from the inside out rather than focusing on the superficial (surface) muscles.

My antics on and off the field are often followed by catchy phrases like Getcha Popcorn Ready or I Loves Me Some Me that keep me motivated. As you begin these workouts, think of your own catchphrases and make them yours; they'll work as affirmation that will keep you pumped.

Let loose, and prepare to entertain your body. It's game day, baby; see you in the end zone!

---

**A Note from Buddy Primm, My Personal Trainer**

This book provides a number of exercises for each muscle group. Why is so much variety necessary? The first reason is that everyone's body is different. An exercise that feels great to me may not feel great to you. The second reason is to combat the number one motivational killer: BOREDOM. The bottom line is that if you perform the same exercises day in and day out, you will eventually become bored. If you become bored, you will not want to exercise. If you change your exercises every two to three months, you will keep your workouts fresh and your motivation level high.

---

When possible, be sure to implement my favorite body adjustment, the pelvic tilt. You'll find tips on how to do this with individual exercises. Even without a professional trainer standing by your side, you will be able to encourage your body to maintain the proper position. The exercises will become more effective, and you will feel better performing them. You can perform each exercise using your T.O. bands, desired free weights, or standard-sized canned food. Note: Some photographs have been shot using Terrell's Home Gym System, the T.O. Strong Man Bands; however, each exercise can be done using alternate forms of resistance, such as dumbbells, canned food, or free weights.

Please note that when using the bands you should be sure to follow the instructions including band setup. When using alternate forms of resistance, follow the instructions minus band setup.

**Why we anchor the bands:** Elastic bands create resistance and tension when you stretch them. In order to stretch the bands, one point needs to be secured or anchored. Anchoring the bands can be achieved by standing on them, wrapping them around a stationary object, or securing them between a door and a door frame with a band-door anchor. Unlike free weights, bands are not bound by gravity and therefore can be anchored at different heights to create tension for many different exercises.

# GENERAL FITNESS: BEGINNER

**Buddy's Tip**  Keep in mind that new exercises will feel awkward the first three or four times you do them. Practice the exercises in front of a mirror; this will help you determine if your form looks similar to the pictures in the book. Practice makes perfect! Stick with it, and before long you will be performing all the exercises like a pro.

## General Information

Perform the exercises in order. Complete the desired number of sets per exercise, and then move on to the next exercise.

## Program Guidelines

**Frequency:**  3 times per week; for example, Monday, Wednesday, and Friday.

**Breathing:**  Learning to use proper breathing techniques is one of the most beneficial things for both short- and long-term physical and emotional health. For the following exercises, we suggest counting to five, inhaling for five on the positive moves, and exhaling for five on the negative move. It is essential to breathe while doing each exercise.

**Warm-up and Cool-down:**  5 minutes of light cardiovascular work: riding an exercise bike, walking on a treadmill, light jogging, or walking in place

**Sets:**  1 per exercise

**Repetitions (Reps) per set: Strength (muscle growth):**  6 to 8 reps

**Strength and musculature (muscle growth and definition):**  8 to 12 reps

**Body toning (muscle definition):**  15 to 18 reps

## Making Progress

Keep in mind that you will need to increase the amount of weight so that you are struggling on the last rep of your targeted rep number. This will ensure that you get the full benefit from every set.

## Exercise 1: Bench Squat

**Muscle group targeted:** Quadriceps and gluteals (front of thighs and buttocks)

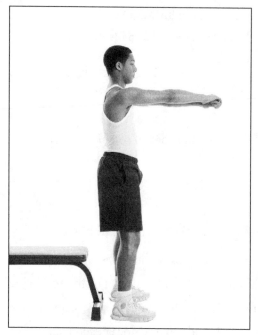

**SETUP/STARTING POSITION:** Sit on the edge of a flat bench or chair with your feet and knees hip-width apart. Your arms should be straight out in front of you, parallel with the floor. Place one hand over the other.

**MOVEMENT:**

**Positive Stage:** Stand up until your body is straight and your legs are almost fully extended.

**Negative Stage:** At a controlled speed, lower your body until your buttocks are once again touching the chair.

> **Buddy's Tip**  Make sure to keep your feet and knees hip-width apart; do not let them push in or bow out.

# Exercise 2: Lying Alternating Lat Pullover

**Muscle group targeted:** Latissimus dorsi (middle and outer back)

**SETUP/STARTING POSITION:** Lie on the floor on your back. Bend your knees and keep your feet flat on the floor. Your knees should be hip-width apart. Reach back over your head and grip a dumbbell in each hand. Rotate your hands so that your palms are facing up. Keep a slight bend in your arms.

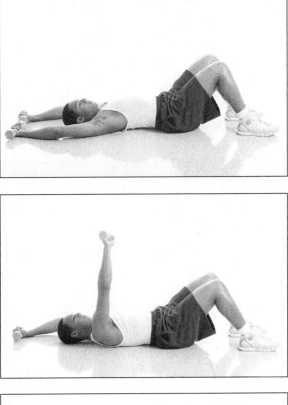

**MOVEMENT:**

**Positive Stage:** Raise your right arm with the weight up and forward until your arm is perpendicular to the floor.

**Negative Stage:** At a controlled speed, lower your arm to the starting position.

Perform the same movement with the left arm. Alternate arms until you complete the desired number of reps.

**ALTERNATIVE RESISTANCE SOURCES:** T.O. resistance bands, standard-sized canned food

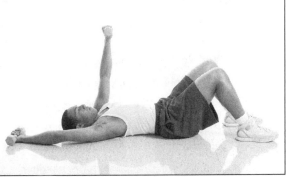

> **Buddy's Tip** Create the pelvic tilt in this lying position by tightening your stomach muscles and pushing your buttocks down toward your feet and up toward the ceiling. Try not to bend your elbow too much when you are raising the weight. Your arm should be almost fully extended.

## Exercise 3. Alternating Seated Lateral Raise

**Muscle group targeted:** Medial deltoid (middle shoulder)

**SETUP/STARTING POSITION:** Grip a dumbbell in each hand and sit on the end of a flat bench. Sit up straight and keep your knees and feet hip-width apart. Your arms should be a few inches out from your sides, slightly bent. Rotate your hands so that your palms are facing behind you.

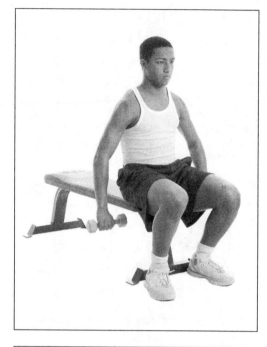

**MOVEMENT:**

**Positive Stage:** Keeping your elbows higher than your hands, raise your right elbow up and out to the side until it is at shoulder height.

**Negative Stage:** At a controlled speed, lower your elbow to the starting position.

Perform the same movement with the left arm. Alternate arms until you complete the desired number of reps.

**ALTERNATIVE RESISTANCE SOURCES:** T.O. resistance bands, standard-sized canned food

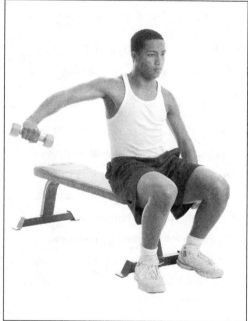

> **Buddy's Tip** Stabilize your lower body with the pelvic tilt. Tighten your abs and push your buttocks forward and upward. As you raise your elbow, relax your shoulder. To help you perform this exercise with the correct form, imagine that you are pouring milk out of a carton as you raise your arm.

# Exercise 4. Lying Biceps Curl

**Muscle group targeted:** Biceps (front of arms)

**SETUP/STARTING POSITION:** Anchor a band at floor level. Sit on the floor, facing the anchor point, and grip a handle in each hand. Lie on your back with your knees bent and your feet flat on the floor. Keep your arms tight to your body and rotate your hands so that your palms are facing up. You should be lying far enough away from the anchor point that there is a slight amount of tension on the band.

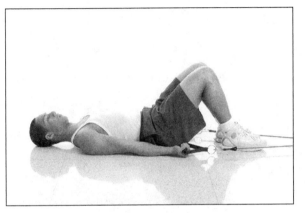

**MOVEMENT:**

**Positive Stage:** Pull the handles and bend your arms until your forearms are perpendicular to the floor.

**Negative Stage:** At a controlled speed, lower the handles to the starting position.

**ALTERNATIVE RESISTANCE SOURCES:** Dumbbells, standard-sized canned food

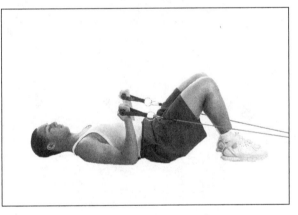

**Buddy's Tip** Stabilize your lower body by creating the pelvic tilt. For this exercise you will need to tighten your stomach muscles and push your buttocks down toward your feet and up toward the ceiling. Your knees should be no wider than hip-width apart. Make sure that your elbows stay firmly on the floor as you curl.

## Exercise 5. Hands-behind-Head Alternating Crunch

**Muscle group targeted:** Rectus abdominus (stomach)

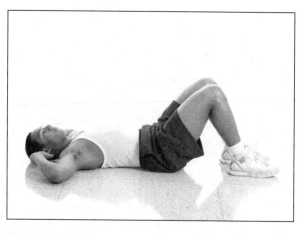

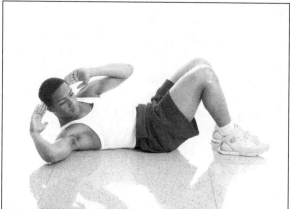

**SETUP/STARTING POSITION:** Lie on your back with your knees bent and your feet flat on the floor. Place your fingertips on the back of your head and push your elbows toward the floor.

**MOVEMENT:**

**Positive Stage:** Raise your left shoulder blade off the floor and move your left elbow toward your right thigh.

**Negative Stage:** When you cannot crunch any higher, slowly lower your left shoulder to the starting position.

Repeat the movement to the other side. Alternate crunches from side to side until you have completed the desired number of reps

**Buddy's Tip** Maintain the pelvic tilt by tightening your stomach muscles and pushing your buttocks down toward your feet and up toward the ceiling. Your knees should be no wider than hip-width apart. Make sure that you do not place your hands too far above your head and pull up from your neck.

## Exercise 6. Lying Triceps Extension

**Muscle group targeted:** Triceps (back of arms)

**SETUP/STARTING POSITION:** Anchor a band at floor level. Lie on your back with your head toward the anchor point. Bend your knees and keep your feet flat on the floor. Reach back and grip a handle in each hand. Position your arms so that your upper arms are perpendicular to and your forearms are parallel with the floor. Keep 12 inches between your elbows. Your hands should be above your forehead with your palms facing in toward each other.

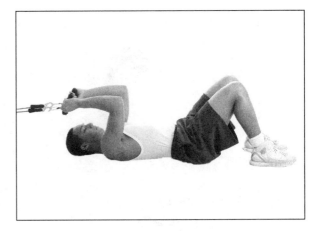

**MOVEMENT:**

**Positive Stage:** Push the handles up and forward until your arms are almost fully extended.

**Negative Stage:** At a controlled speed, lower the handles to the starting position.

**ALTERNATIVE RESISTANCE SOURCES:** Dumbbells, standard-sized canned food

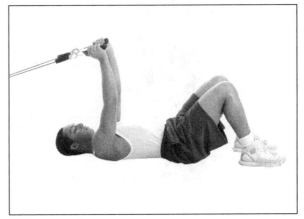

**Buddy's Tip** Create the pelvic tilt for this exercise by tightening your stomach muscles and pushing your buttocks toward your feet and up toward the ceiling. Your knees should be no wider than hip-width apart. Keep your elbows stationary, in the same position. If they move forward or backward during the exercise, you will begin to use other muscle groups instead of your triceps.

## Exercise 7. Wall Push-up

**Muscle group targeted:** Pectoralis major (chest)

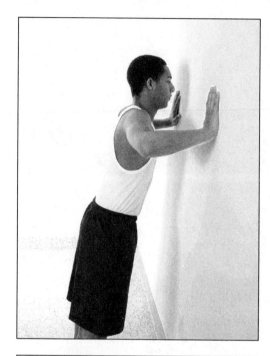

**SETUP/STARTING POSITION:** Stand up straight facing a sturdy wall. Your toes should be about 2½ feet away from the wall. Lean forward and place your palms on the wall with your thumbs facing inward. Position your arms so that your elbows are at shoulder height and your hands are a few inches more than shoulder-width apart.

**MOVEMENT:**

**Positive Stage:** Press your body back until your hands are no longer touching the wall.

**Negative Stage:** When you are standing almost straight, let gravity slowly draw your body forward until you are back at the starting position.

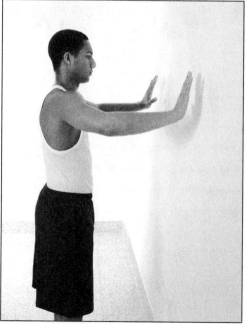

> **Buddy's Tip** Implement the pelvic tilt for this exercise by tightening your stomach muscles and pushing your buttocks forward and upward. Keep your elbows up at shoulder height.

# GENERAL FITNESS: INTERMEDIATE

## General Information
Perform the exercises in order. Complete the desired number of sets per exercise, and then move on to the next exercise.

## Program Guidelines
**Frequency:**  3 times per week: for example, Monday, Wednesday, and Friday

**Warm-up and cool-down:**  5 minutes of light cardiovascular work: riding an exercise bike, walking on a treadmill, light jogging, or walking in place

**Sets:**  2 per exercise

**Repetitions (reps) per set:**  Strength: 6 to 8 reps

**Strength and musculature:**  8 to 12 reps

**Body toning:**  15 to 18 reps

**Rep speed:**  Use a 1 count (say "one-Mississippi" in your head) during the positive stage of the movement and again during the negative stage.

**Breathing:**  Be sure to breathe during the exercises: specifically, exhale during the positive stage of the movement.

## Making Progress
Keep in mind that you will need to adjust the resistance so that you are struggling on the last rep of your targeted rep number. This will ensure that you get the full benefit from every set.

## Exercise 1. Dumbbell-Tight-to-Chest Squat

**Muscle group targeted:** Quadriceps and gluteals (thighs and buttocks)

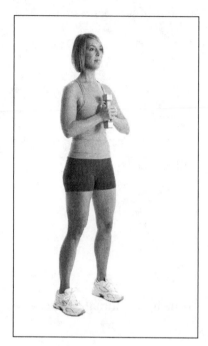

**SETUP/STARTING POSITION:** Bend down and grip a dumbbell with two hands. Stand up straight with your feet hip-width apart and your knees slightly bent. Hold the dumbbell tight to your chest. Your arms should be tight to your sides with your elbows down. Keep your chest up and your head straight.

**MOVEMENT:**

**Positive Stage:** Push from your heels and raise your body to the starting position.

**Negative Stage:** At a controlled speed, lower your body and squat down until your legs stop naturally.

**ALTERNATIVE RESISTANCE SOURCES:**

Resistance bands, standard-sized canned food

**Buddy's Tip** Do not let your knees move too far forward during the exercise. The rule of thumb is that your kneecaps should not move forward past your toes as you squat.

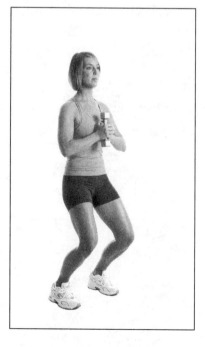

## Exercise 2. Lying Two-Arm Lat Pullover

**Muscle group targeted:** Latissimus dorsi (middle and outer back)

**SETUP/STARTING POSITION:** Anchor a band at floor level. Lie on your back with your knees bent and your feet flat on the floor. Reach back over your head and grip a handle in each hand. Rotate your hands so that your palms are facing up. Keep a slight bend in your arms.

**MOVEMENT:**

**Positive Stage:** Push the handles up and forward until your arms are perpendicular to the floor.

**Negative Stage:** At a controlled speed, lower the handles to the starting position.

**ALTERNATIVE RESISTANCE SOURCES:** Dumbbells, standard-sized canned food

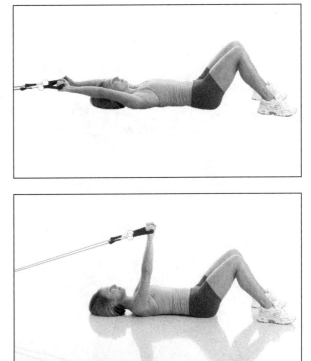

> **Buddy's Tip** Create the pelvic tilt in this lying position by tightening your stomach muscles and pushing your buttocks down toward your feet and up toward the ceiling. Try not to bend your elbows too much when you are raising the weight. Your arms should be almost fully extended. Also, keep your hands shoulder-width apart.

## Exercise 3. Cross-Legged Push-up

**Muscle group targeted:** Pectoralis major (chest)

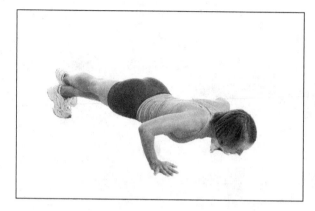

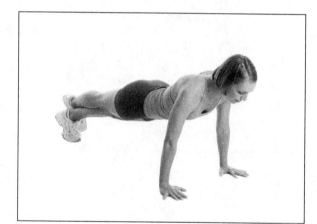

**SETUP/STARTING POSITION:** Lie facedown on the floor with your legs straight and one leg crossed over the other. Position your arms straight out to the sides with your hands directly under your elbows. Now push up so that your chest is 3 to 4 inches off the floor.

**MOVEMENT:**

**Positive Stage:** Keeping your head straight, push from your palms and raise your body until your arms are almost fully extended.

**Negative Stage:** At a controlled speed, lower your body to the starting position.

**Buddy's Tip** Before you push up for the first rep, make sure your pelvis is in the right position. To create the pelvic tilt, tighten your stomach muscles and push your buttocks down toward the floor and up toward your head. Do not let your midsection droop as you push your body off the floor. A side view should show your body straight as a board.

# Exercise 4. Seated Shoulder Press

**Muscle group targeted:** Anterior deltoid (front shoulder)

**SETUP/STARTING POSITION:** Grip a dumbbell in each hand and sit on the end of a flat bench. Keep your knees and feet shoulder-width apart. Position your arms so that your upper arms are parallel with the floor and your forearms are perpendicular. Your elbows should be back.

**MOVEMENT:**

**Positive Stage:** Push the weights up and together over your head until your arms are almost fully extended.

**Negative Stage:** At a controlled speed, lower the weights to the starting position.

**ALTERNATIVE RESISTANCE SOURCES:** T.O. Resistance bands, standard-sized canned food

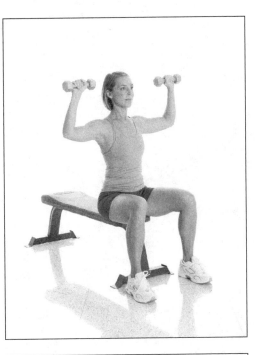

> **Buddy's Tip** Create the pelvic tilt in this seated position by tightening your stomach muscles and pushing your buttocks forward and upward.

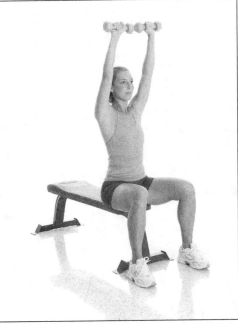

## Exercise 5. Seated Alternating Hammer Curl

**Muscle group targeted:** Biceps (front of arms)

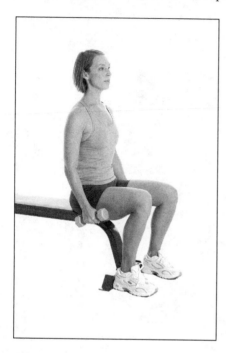

**SETUP/STARTING POSITION:** Grip a dumbbell in each hand and sit on the end of a flat bench. Keep your knees and feet shoulder-width apart. Your arms should be tight to your body and perpendicular to the floor. Keep your elbows stationary at your sides, with a slight bend. Rotate your hands so that your palms are facing in toward your outer thighs.

**MOVEMENT:**

**Positive Stage:** Raise the right handle until your right forearm is a little higher than parallel with the floor.

**Negative Stage:** At a controlled speed, lower the weight to the starting position.

Perform the same movement with the left arm. Alternate arms until you complete the desired number of reps.

**ALTERNATIVE RESISTANCE SOURCES:** T.O Resistance bands, standard-sized canned food

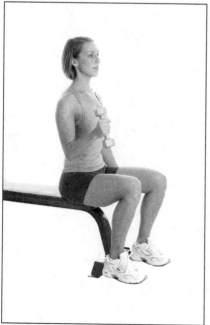

> **Buddy's Tip** Stabilize your body with the pelvic tilt. Tighten your stomach muscles and push your buttocks forward and upward. Be sure to keep your elbow stationary as your raise the weight.

# Exercise 6. Knees-up, Hands-to-Sky Crunches

**Muscle group targeted:** Rectus abdominus (stomach)

**SETUP/STARTING POSITION:** Lie on your back. Lift your feet and position your legs so that your thighs are perpendicular to the floor and your calves are parallel. Raise your arms straight up so that they are perpendicular to the floor and almost fully extended.

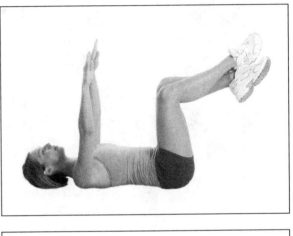

**MOVEMENT:**

**Positive Stage:** Lift your shoulder blades off the floor and crunch up until you cannot crunch any higher.

**Negative Stage:** At a controlled speed, lower your shoulder blades to the starting position.

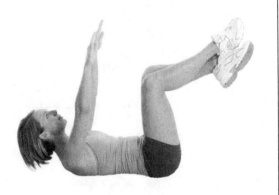

> **Buddy's Tip**  To perform this crunch correctly, keep your head straight and move your hands straight up toward the ceiling.

## Exercise 7. Two-Arm Triceps Kickback

**Muscle group targeted:** Triceps (back of arm)

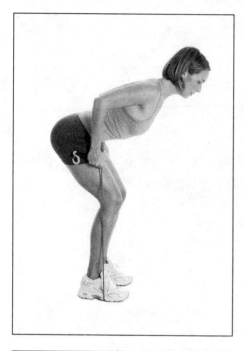

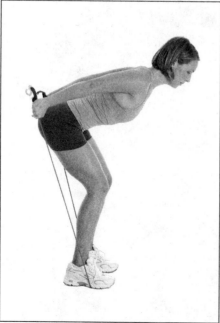

**SETUP/STARTING POSITION:** Start by standing with your feet hip-width apart on a band. Make sure that the length of the band from the outside of your shoe to the handle is the same on both sides. Reach down and grip the band right below the clip (or handle). Position your body so that your buttocks are sticking out and your upper body is leaning forward. Create a slight arch in your back and bend your knees. Raise your arms so that your upper arms are parallel with the floor and your forearms are perpendicular. The palms of your hands should be rotated in, facing your outer thighs.

**MOVEMENT:**

**Positive Stage:** Push both hands back behind you until your arms are almost fully extended.

**Negative Stage:** At a controlled speed, lower your hands to the starting position.

**ALTERNATIVE RESISTANCE SOURCES:** Dumbbells, standard-sized canned food

**Buddy's Tip** Keep your arms tight to your body. Your elbows should stay stationary; they should not move up or down as you straighten your arms.

# GENERAL FITNESS: ADVANCED

> **Buddy's Tip** The advanced general fitness routine is intended for individuals who are already at an advanced level or who have worked their way up from the previous routines. I train hundreds of athletes who are at the advanced level, and I know that it can be easy to focus on using higher amounts of resistance, but you should also continue to focus on your form. More is not always better; I want you to train smart, not just hard.
>
> It is important, especially at this level of training, to implement the pelvic tilt by tightening your stomach muscles and pulling your buttocks forward toward the ceiling and up toward your head. We want your body to be superbly conditioned without pain and without injury.

## General Information

Perform the exercises in order. Complete the desired number of sets per exercise, and then move on to the next exercise.

## Program Guidelines

**Frequency:** 3 times per week; for example, Monday, Wednesday, and Friday

**Warm-up and cool-down:** 5 minutes of light cardiovascular work: riding an exercise bike, walking on a treadmill, light jogging, or walking in place

**Sets:** 3 per exercise

**Repetitions (reps) per set:** Strength: 6 to 8 reps

**Strength and musculature:** 8 to 12 reps

**Body toning:** 15 to 18 reps

**Rep speed:** Use a 1 count (say "one-Mississippi" in your head) during the positive stage of the movement and again during the negative stage.

**Breathing:** Be sure to exhale during the positive stage of the movement.

## Making Progress

You will need to adjust the resistance so that you are struggling on the last rep of your targeted rep number to ensure that you get the full benefit from every set.

## Exercise 1. Lying Bench Leg Curl

**Muscle group targeted:** Hamstrings (back of legs)

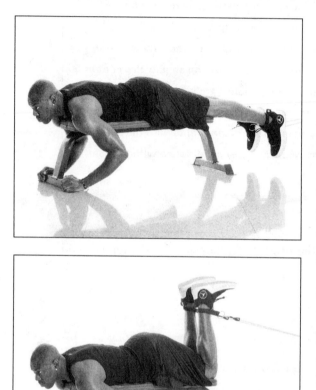

**SETUP/STARTING POSITION:** Face away from the anchor point of your bands and attach each end to an ankle strap. Lie facedown on a bench and position your body so that your knees are at the end of the bench. The bench should be far enough away from the anchor point so that there is a slight amount of tension on the band. Stabilize your body by gripping the bench or placing your hands on the floor. Keep your head down. This is a fundamental hamstring exercise, and it works!

**MOVEMENT:**

**Positive Stage:** Keeping your knees and feet hip-width apart, bend your legs and move your heels toward your buttocks until your legs stop bending naturally.

**Negative Stage:** At a controlled speed, lower your legs to the starting position.

**ALTERNATIVE RESISTANCE SOURCE:** Ankle weights

**Buddy's Tip** Create a pelvic tilt by tightening the stomach muscles and pulling the buttocks down toward the floor and up toward your head. If you feel that you are tightening your calves as you bend your legs, point your toes; this will disengage the calves and help isolate the hamstrings.

## Exercise 2. Bench Press

**Muscle group targeted:** pectoralis major (chest)

**SETUP/STARTING POSITION:** Grip a dumbbell in each hand and sit on the edge of a flat bench. Lie back and move your body so that your head is at the end of the bench. Keep your arms tight to your body with your hands just over your chest. Rotate your wrists so that your palms are facing in toward each other. Your knees and feet should be hip-width apart.

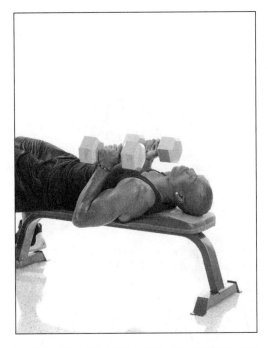

**MOVEMENT:**

**Positive Stage:** Press the dumbbells straight up until your arms are almost fully extended.

**Negative Stage:** At a controlled speed, lower the weights to the starting position.

**ALTERNATIVE RESISTANCE SOURCES:** T.O. Resistance bands, standard-sized canned food

> **Buddy's Tip** Create the pelvic tilt for this exercise by tightening the stomach muscles and pushing your buttocks down toward your feet and up toward the ceiling. As you press the weights up, keep your hands 12 inches apart.

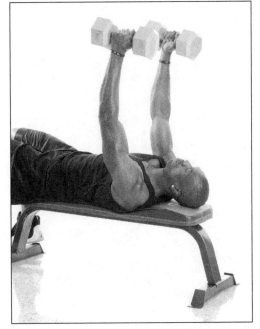

## Exercise 3. Seated Lateral Raises

**Muscle group targeted:** Medial deltoid (side shoulder)

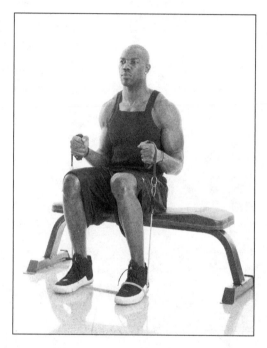

**SETUP/STARTING POSITION:** Sit on a flat bench with your feet hip-width apart. Step on a band with one foot and wrap it once around the other. Make sure that the length of the band from the outside of your shoe to the handle is the same on both sides. With a handle in each hand, sit up straight. Keep your arms at your sides, bent at a 90-degree angle. Your palms should be facing in toward each other.

**MOVEMENT:**

**Positive Stage:** Keeping your elbows higher than your hands, raise your elbows up and out to the side until they are at shoulder height.

**Negative Stage:** At a controlled speed, lower your elbows to the starting position.

**ALTERNATIVE RESISTANCE SOURCES:** Dumbbells, standard-sized canned food

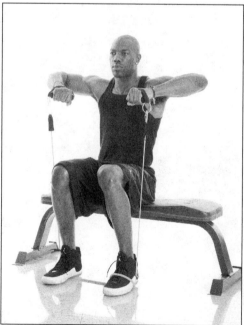

> **Buddy's Tip** As you raise your elbows, relax your shoulders. To help you perform this exercise with the correct form, imagine that you are pouring milk out of cartons as you raise your arms.

# Exercise 4. One-arm Bent-over Row

**Muscle group targeted:** Latissimus dorsi (upper and outer back)

**SETUP/STARTING POSITION:** Stand at the end of a flat bench and place your right foot forward against the edge of the bench and your left foot back. Wrap a band once around your right foot so that there is 6 inches of elastic between the outside of your shoe and a handle. Place your left hand on the end of the bench for support. Keep your head straight, looking forward. Your feet should be no wider than hip-width apart.

**MOVEMENT:**

**Positive Stage:** Pull the handle up and back until your hand is by your hip.

**Negative Stage:** At a controlled speed, lower the handle to the starting position.

**ALTERNATIVE RESISTANCE SOURCES:** Dumbbells, standard-sized canned food

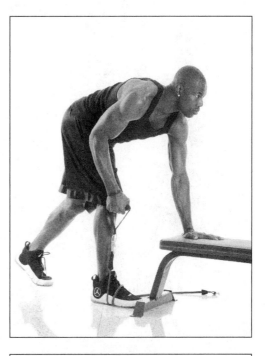

**Buddy's Tip**  To help you use the proper form, imagine that you are placing a coin in your back pocket. To isolate the back muscles, keep a closed but loose grip on the handle.

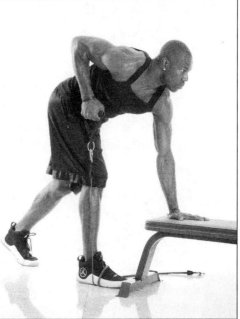

## Exercise 5. Water Ski Squat

**Muscle group targeted:** Quadriceps and gluteus maximus (thighs and buttocks)

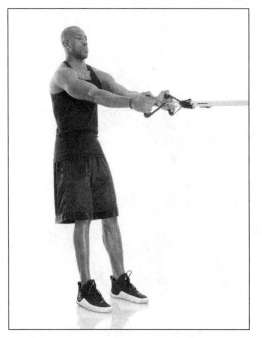

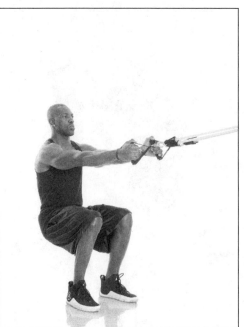

**SETUP/STARTING POSITION:** Anchor a band at chest height. Position your body so that you are facing the anchor point, and grip a handle in each hand. Hold your arms straight out in front of you 6 inches apart and parallel with the floor. Move back so that there is a good amount of tension on the band. Keep your feet and knees hip-width apart. Your knees should be slightly bent.

**MOVEMENT:**

**Negative Stage:** At a controlled speed, squat down until your thighs are parallel with the floor.

**Positive Stage:** Push up until you are back to the starting position.

**ALTERNATIVE RESISTANCE SOURCE:** Towel or jump rope to wrap around a stationary object, such as a door hinge.

**Buddy's Tip** As you lower your body, mimic the motion of sitting in a chair. You should actually be squatting back as well as down. This will ensure that your legs are in the proper position. Try not to let your knees push in or bow out; keep them hip-width apart.

# Exercise 6. Standing Hammer Curls

**Muscle group targeted:** Biceps (front of arms)

**SETUP/STARTING POSITION:** Stand with your feet hip-width apart on a band. Make sure that the length of the band from the outside of your shoe to the handle is the same on both sides. Reach down and grip an ankle strap (or handle) in each hand. Stand up straight with your arms at your sides and your palms resting against your outer thighs. Keep your knees slightly bent and lean forward a little.

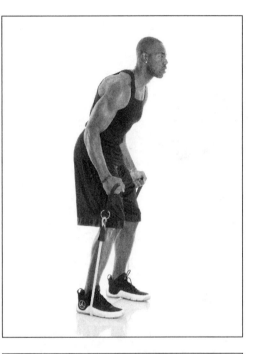

**MOVEMENT:**

**Positive Stage:** Raise the ankle straps forward and up until they are at chest height.

**Negative Stage:** At a controlled speed, lower the ankle straps to the starting position.

**ALTERNATIVE RESISTANCE SOURCES:** Dumbbells, standard-sized canned food

> **Buddy's Tip** Stabilize your body by tightening your stomach muscles and pushing your buttocks forward and upward. Keep your elbows stationary at your sides; they should not move forward or backward as your raise the ankle straps. If you are unable to keep your elbows stationary, try using less tension.

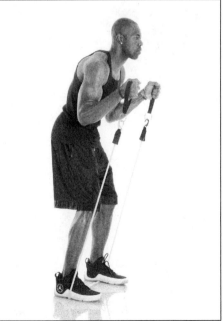

## Exercise 7. Resisted Abdominal Crunch

**Muscle group targeted:** Rectus abdominus (stomach)

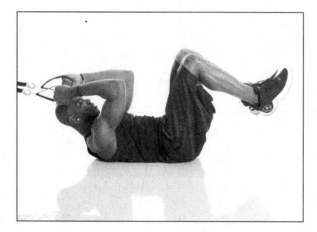

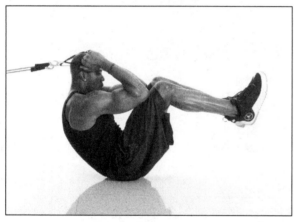

**SETUP/STARTING POSITION:** Anchor a band at knee height. Sit down with your back to the anchor point. Lie back and grip an ankle strap (or handle) with each hand. Move your body away from the anchor point so that there is a slight amount of tension on the band. Position your hands just above your forehead with your palms facing in. Your elbows should have 6 inches between them. Raise your feet 12 inches and keep your thighs parallel with the floor.

**MOVEMENT:**

**Positive Stage:** Raise your shoulders off the floor and crunch up until your elbows touch your knees.

**Negative Stage:** At a controlled speed, lower your shoulders to the starting position.

**ALTERNATIVE RESISTANCE SOURCES:** Dumbbells, standard-sized canned food

**Buddy's Tip** Before you perform the first crunch, implement the pelvic tilt: tighten your stomach muscles and push your buttocks toward your feet and up toward the ceiling.

# BODY TONING: BEGINNER

## General Information

This body-toning workout is designed as an exercise circuit, one of the best ways to tone your muscles quickly and effectively. Perform the exercises and cardio moves in order. When you have completed the last exercise, you have completed one circuit.

## Program Guidelines

**Frequency:** 3 to 5 times per week

**Warm-up:** 5 minutes of light cardiovascular exercise: riding an exercise bike, walking on a treadmill, doing jumping jacks, jogging, or walking in place

**Estimated workout time per circuit:** 10 minutes, not including the warm-up and cool-down

**Repetitions (reps):** 15 per exercise

**Rep speed:** Use a 1 count (say "one-Mississippi" in your head) during the positive stage of the movement and a 1 count (say "one-Mississippi") during the negative stage.

**Cardio moves:** There are three cardio moves for this body-toning routine:

1. Walking in place

2. Stepping from side to side

3. Doing jumping jacks with hands on hips

**Breathing:** Keep breathing during the exercises and cardio segments.

**Cool-down:** 5 minutes of light cardiovascular exercise: riding an exercise bike, walking on a treadmill, doing jumping jacks, jogging, or walking in place

## Making Progress

After completing one full circuit, see how you feel. If you can, try to complete another two circuits. When you are able to complete three circuits in a row easily, it is time to move up to the intermediate body-toning routine. Your ultimate goal is to complete three consecutive full circuits of the advanced body-toning program.

## Exercise 1. Squat with Hands on Thighs

(see page 70 for photo example)

**Muscle group targeted:** Quadriceps and gluteus maximus (thighs and buttocks)

**SETUP/STARTING POSITION:** Stand up straight with your feet facing forward. Place the palms of your hands on the top of your thighs. Keep your knees slightly bent and your chest up.

**MOVEMENT:**

**Negative Stage:** Lower your body until your thighs are parallel with the floor.

**Positive Stage:** Push from your heels and raise your body to the starting position.

> **Buddy's Tip** Start the negative stage of the movement by sticking out your buttocks, similar to the motion required for sitting in a chair. Make sure that your knees are not pushing in toward each other or bowing out. If you need extra assistance raising your body during the positive stage of the movement, use your arms to push off from your thighs.

Perform one of the three specified cardio moves for 30 seconds.

# Exercise 2. Alternating Standing One-Arm Back Row

**Muscle group targeted:** Latissimus dorsi (middle and outer back)

**SETUP/STARTING POSITION:** Lay a band horizontally on the floor in front of you. Step on the band with one foot and wrap it once around the other. Make sure that the length of the band from the outside of your shoe to the handle is the same on the both sides. Grip a handle in each hand. Stand up straight, with your knees slightly bent. Your arms should be straight down, with your palms resting against your outer thighs.

**MOVEMENT:**

**Positive Stage:** Pull the right handle up and back until it is next to your right hip.

**Negative Stage:** At a controlled speed, lower the handle forward and down until it is back to the starting position.

Perform the same movement with the left arm. Alternate arms until you complete the desired number of reps.

**ALTERNATIVE RESISTANCE SOURCES:** Dumbbells, standard-sized canned food

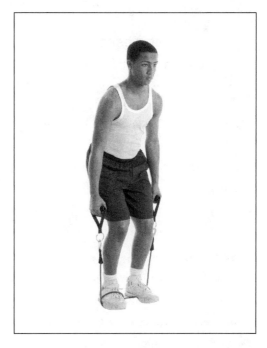

**Buddy's Tip** To create the proper form while you are pulling, imagine that you are placing a coin in your back pocket. To help isolate your back muscles, keep a closed but loose grip on the handle.

Perform one of the three specified cardio moves for 30 seconds.

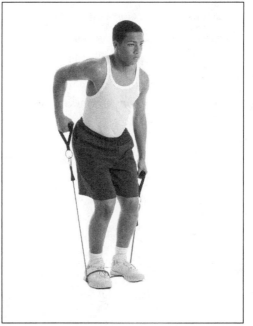

## Exercise 3. Lunge, Hands on Thighs

(see page 72 for photo example)

**Muscle group targeted:** Quadriceps and gluteus maximus (thighs and buttocks)

**SETUP/STARTING POSITION:** Stand up straight with your left foot forward. Place both hands on top of your left thigh. Your left knee should be slightly bent.

**MOVEMENT:**

**Negative Stage:** Keeping your chest up, lower your body until your left leg is parallel with the floor.

**Positive Stage:** Push from your heel and raise your body until your left leg is back at the starting position.

Complete the desired number of reps and switch sides.

> **Buddy's Tip** The knee of your front leg should not move forward during the exercise. The rule of thumb is that your front knee should be directly above the toes of your front foot. If you need extra assistance raising your body during the positive stage of the movement, use your arms to push off from your thigh.

Perform one of the three specified cardio moves for 30 seconds.

# Exercise 4. Alternating Kneeling One-arm Triceps Extension

**Muscle group targeted:** Triceps (back of arm)

**SETUP/STARTING POSITION:** Grip the handle of a band in each hand and hang the band down in front of your ankles. Keeping the band at ankle height, kneel down so that both knees are on the floor. Raise the handles so that your hands are behind your head and about 12 inches apart. Your elbows should be in and up. Rotate your hands so that your palms are facing in toward each other.

**MOVEMENT:**

**Positive Stage:** Push your left hand straight up until your arm is almost fully extended.

**Negative Stage:** At a controlled speed, lower your hand to the starting position.

Perform the same movement with the right arm. Alternate arms until you complete the desired number of reps.

**ALTERNATIVE RESISTANCE SOURCES:** Dumbbells, standard-sized canned food

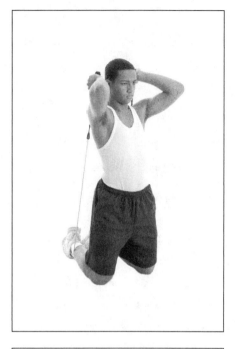

> **Buddy's Tip** Create the pelvic tilt for this exercise by tightening your stomach muscles and pushing your buttocks forward and upward. It is very important that you keep your elbows up as you push.

Perform one of the three specified cardio moves for 30 seconds.

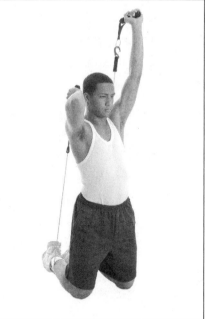

## Exercise 5. Hammer Curl

(see page 74 for photo example)

**Muscle group targeted:** Biceps (front of arms)

**SETUP/STARTING POSITION:** Stand up straight with your feet hip-width apart. Keep your arms down at your sides with your palms resting on your outer thighs. Keep your knees slightly bent and your head straight.

**MOVEMENT:**

**Positive Stage:** Raise your hands forward and up until they are at chest height.

**Negative Stage:** At a controlled speed, lower your hands to the starting position.

**ALTERNATIVE RESISTANCE SOURCES:** Dumbbells, standard-sized canned food

> **Buddy's Tip** Implement the pelvic tilt for this exercise by tightening your stomach muscles and pushing your buttocks forward and upward. Keep your elbows stationary at your sides. Do not move your elbows forward or back as you raise your hands.

Perform one of the three specified cardio moves for 30 seconds.

## Exercise 6. Standing Lateral Raise

(see page 75 for photo example)

**Muscle group targeted:** Medial deltoid (side shoulder)

**SETUP/STARTING POSITION:** Stand up straight with your knees and feet hip-width apart. Keep your arms at your sides and your palms facing in toward each other. Keep your knees slightly bent.

**MOVEMENT:**

**Positive Stage:** Raise your arms straight out to the side until your elbows reach shoulder height.

**Negative Stage:** At a controlled speed, lower your arms to the starting position

---

**Buddy's Tip** Before you start the movement, create the pelvic tilt by tightening your stomach muscles and pulling your buttocks forward and upward. Keep your elbows higher than your hands as your raise your arms. A great trick to help you use proper form is to imagine that you are pouring milk out of cartons as you raise your arms.

---

Perform one of the three specified cardio moves for 30 seconds.

## Exercise 7. Bent-Leg Push-up

(see page 76 for photo example)

**Muscle group targeted:** Pectoralis major (chest)

**SETUP/STARTING POSITION:** Lie facedown on the floor with your knees bent and toes up, about 2 feet off the floor. Position your arms straight out to the sides with your hands directly under your elbows.

**MOVEMENT:**

**Positive Stage:** Keeping your head straight, push from your palms and raise your chest off the floor until your arms are almost fully extended.

**Negative Stage:** At a controlled speed, lower your body to the starting position.

> **Buddy's Tip** Before you push up against the resistance for the first rep, make sure your pelvis is in the right position. To create the right position, tighten your stomach muscles and pull your buttocks down toward the floor and up toward your head.

# Exercise 8. Superman Alternating Back Extension

(see page 77 for photo example)

**Muscle group targeted:**  Erector spinae (lower back)

**SETUP/STARTING POSITION:**  Lie facedown on the floor with your arms extended straight over your head and your legs straight. Keep your hands and feet a few inches more than shoulder-width apart. Place your palms flat on the floor.

**MOVEMENT:**

**Positive Stage:**  Simultaneously raise your right arm and left thigh 2 to 3 inches off the floor.

**Negative Stage:**  At a controlled speed, lower your arm and leg to the starting position.

Perform the same movement with the left arm and right thigh. Alternate arms and legs until you complete the desired number of reps.

> **Buddy's Tip**  This is a great beginner exercise for strengthening your lower back. It may take some time to master. However, a strong lower back will help with almost every other exercise listed in this book.

## Exercise 9. Hands-Toward-Feet Crunches

(see page 78 for photo example)

**Muscle group targeted:** Rectus abdominus (stomach)

**SETUP/STARTING POSITION:** Lie on your back with your knees bent and your feet flat on the floor. Your arms should be straight and on the floor, tight to your body. Rotate your hands so that your palms are on the floor.

**MOVEMENT:**

**Positive Stage:** Keeping your chin tucked in, raise your shoulder blades off the floor, moving your hands toward your feet.

**Negative Stage:** When you feel as though you cannot move your hands any farther, slowly lower your shoulder blades and hands to the starting position.

> **Buddy's Tip** Remember to exhale during the positive stage and inhale during the negative stage of this exercise.

# BODY TONING: INTERMEDIATE

## Program Guidelines

**Frequency:**  3 to 5 times per week

**Warm-up:**  5 minutes of light cardiovascular exercise: riding an exercise bike, walking on a treadmill, doing jumping jacks, jogging, or walking in place

**Estimated workout time per circuit:**  10 minutes, not including the warm-up and cool-down

**Repetitions (reps):**  18 per exercise

**Rep speed:**  Use a 1 count (say "one-Mississippi" in your head) during the positive stage of the movement and again during the negative stage.

**Cardio moves:**  There are three cardio moves for this body-toning routine:

1. Doing jumping jacks

2. Jogging in place

3. Jumping rope without a rope

**Breathing:**  Keep breathing during the exercises and cardio segments.

**Cool-down:**  5 minutes of light cardiovascular exercise:  riding an exercise bike, walking on a treadmill, jumping jacks, jogging, or walking in place

## Making Progress

After completing one full circuit, see how you feel. If you can, try to complete another two circuits. When you are able to complete three intermediate body-toning circuits in a row easily, it is time to move up to the advanced body-toning routine. Your ultimate goal over time is to complete three consecutive full circuits of the advanced body-toning program.

## Exercise 1. Squat with Hands on Thighs

(see page 70 for photo example)

**Muscle group targeted:** Quadriceps and gluteus maximus (thighs and buttocks)

**SETUP/STARTING POSITION:** Stand on a band with your feet shoulder-width apart, and pointing forward. Make sure that the length of the band from the outside of your shoe to the handle is the same on both sides. Bend down and grip a handle in each hand. Place the palms of your hands on the top of your thighs. Keep your knees slightly bent and your chest up.

**MOVEMENT:**

**Negative Stage:** Lower your body until your thighs are parallel with the floor.

**Positive Stage:** Push from your heels and raise your body the starting position.

> **Buddy's Tip** This is an incredible exercise for strengthening and shaping the entire leg. It will take some practice to master, so don't give up! Start the negative stage of the movement by sticking out your buttocks, similar to the motion required for sitting in a chair. Make sure that your knees are not pushing in toward each other or bowing out. If this is the case, decrease the resistance.

Perform one of the three specified cardio moves for 30 seconds.

# Exercise 2. Standing Two-Arm Back Row

**Muscle group targeted:** Latissimus dorsi (middle and outer back)

**SETUP/STARTING POSITION:** Lay a band on the floor in front of you. Step on the band with one foot and wrap it once around the other. Make sure that the length of the band from the outside of your shoe to the handle is the same on both sides. Grip a handle in each hand. Position your body so that your buttocks are sticking out and your upper body is leaning forward. Create a slight arch in your back, and bend your knees. Your arms should be straight down and tight to your body. Rotate your hands so that your palms are turned in, resting against your outer thighs.

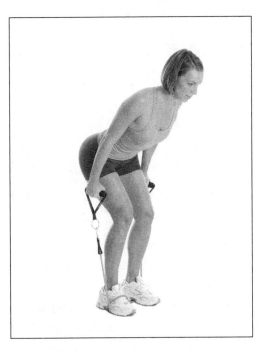

**MOVEMENT:**

**Positive Stage:** Pull the handles up and back until they are next to your hips.

**Negative Stage:** At a controlled speed, lower the handles forward and down until they are at the starting position.

**ALTERNATIVE RESISTANCE SOURCES:** Dumbbells, standard-sized canned food

> **Buddy's Tip** To create the proper form while you are pulling, imagine that you are placing coins in your back pockets. To help isolate your back muscles, keep a closed but loose grip on the handle.

Perform one of the three specified cardio moves for 30 seconds.

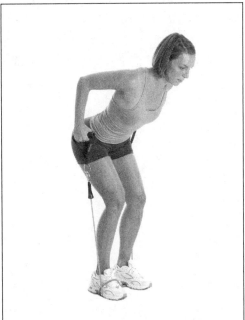

## Exercise 3. Lunge

(see page 72 for photo example)

**Muscle group targeted:** Quadriceps and gluteus maximus (thighs and buttocks)

**SETUP/STARTING POSITION:** Stand up straight with your left foot forward. Raise your hands to shoulder height and rotate your palms so that they are facing forward. Your left knee should be slightly bent.

**MOVEMENT:**

**Negative Stage:** Keeping your chest up, lower your body until your left leg is parallel with the floor.

**Positive Stage:** Push from your heel and raise your body until your left leg is back at the starting position.

Complete the desired number of reps and then switch sides.

---

**Buddy's Tip** The knee of your front leg should not move forward during the exercise. The rule of thumb is that your front knee should be directly above the toes of your front foot.

---

Perform one of the three specified cardio moves for 30 seconds.

## Exercise 4. Kneeling Two-Arm Triceps Extension

**Muscle group targeted:** Triceps (back of arms)

**SETUP/STARTING POSITION:** Grip the handle of a band in each hand and hang the band down in front of your ankles. Keeping the band at ankle height, kneel down so that both knees are on the floor. Raise the handles so that your hands are behind your head and about 12 inches apart. Your elbows should be in and up. Rotate your hands so that your palms are facing in toward each other.

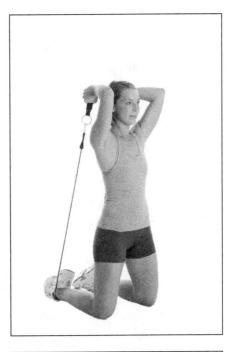

**MOVEMENT:**

**Positive Stage:** Push your hands straight up until your arms are almost fully extended.

**Negative Stage:** At a controlled speed, lower your hands to the starting position.

**ALTERNATIVE RESISTANCE SOURCES:** Dumbbells, standard-sized canned food

> **Buddy's Tip** Create the pelvic tilt for this exercise by tightening your stomach muscles and pushing your buttocks forward and upward. It is very important that you keep your elbows up and shoulder-width apart as you push.

Perform one of the three specified cardio moves for 30 seconds.

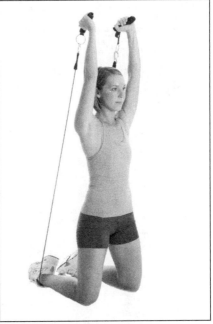

## Exercise 5. Alternating Hammer Curl

(see page 74 for photo example)

**Muscle group targeted:** Biceps (front of arms)

**SETUP/STARTING POSITION:** Grip a dumbbell in each hand and stand up straight with your feet hip-width apart. Keep your arms down at your sides with your palms resting on your outer thighs. Keep your knees slightly bent and your head straight.

**MOVEMENT:**

**Positive Stage:** Raise your right hand forward and up until it is at chest height.

**Negative Stage:** At a controlled speed, lower your right hand until it is back at the starting position.

Switch arms and curl with the left hand. Alternate arms until you complete the desired number of reps.

**ALTERNATIVE RESISTANCE SOURCES:** T.O. Resistance bands, standard-sized canned food

> **Buddy's Tip** Create the pelvic tilt for this exercise by tightening your stomach muscles and pushing your buttocks forward and upward. Keep your elbows stationary at your sides. Do not move your elbows forward or back as you raise the dumbbells.

Perform one of the three specified cardio moves for 30 seconds.

## Exercise 6. Standing Alternating Lateral Raise

(see page 75 for photo example)

**Muscle group targeted:** Medial deltoid (side shoulder)

**SETUP/STARTING POSITION:** Stand on a band with your feet hip-width apart. Make sure that the length of the band from the outside of your shoe to the handle is the same on both sides. Reach down and grip a handle in each hand. Stand up straight with your arms at your sides and your palms facing in toward each other. Keep your knees slightly bent.

**MOVEMENT:**

**Positive Stage:** Raise your right arm straight out to the side until your elbow reaches shoulder height.

**Negative Stage:** At a controlled speed, lower your right arm to the starting position.

Switch arms and raise only your left arm. Alternate arms until you complete the desired number of reps.

**ALTERNATIVE RESISTANCE SOURCES:**

Dumbbells, standard-sized canned food

---

**Buddy's Tip** Before you start the movement, create the pelvic tilt by tightening your stomach muscles and pulling your buttocks forward and upward. Keep your elbows higher than your hands as you raise your arms. A great trick to help you use proper form is to imagine that you are pouring milk out of cartons as you raise your arms.

---

Perform one of the three specified cardio moves for 30 seconds.

## Exercise 7. Push-up

(see page 76 for photo example)

**Muscle group targeted:**  Pectoralis major (chest)

**SETUP/STARTING POSITION:**  Lie facedown on the floor with your legs straight. Position your arms straight out to the sides with your hands directly under your elbows.

**MOVEMENT:**

**Positive Stage:**  Keeping your head straight, push from your palms and raise your body off the floor until your arms are almost fully extended.

**Negative Stage:**  At a controlled speed, lower your body to the starting position.

> **Buddy's Tip**  Before you push up against the resistance for the first rep, make sure your pelvis is in the right position. To create the right position, tighten your stomach muscles and pull your buttocks down toward the floor and up toward your head. Do not let your midsection droop as you push your body off the floor. A side view of your body should show your body straight as a board.

## Exercise 8. Superman Back Extension (Upper Body Only)

(see page 77 for photo example)

**Muscle group targeted:** Erector spinae (lower back)

**SETUP/STARTING POSITION:** Lie facedown on the floor with your arms extended straight over your head and your legs straight. Keep your hands 2 to 3 inches more than shoulder-width apart. Place your palms flat on the floor.

**MOVEMENT:**

**Positive Stage:** Raise your chest 2 to 3 inches off the floor.

**Negative Stage:** At a controlled speed, lower your chest to the starting position.

> **Buddy's Tip** For those of you who need to strengthen your lower back, this is a supereffective and safe exercise. It may take some time to master. As you raise your upper body off the ground, keep your head straight at the same level as your arms.

## Exercise 9. Hands-Up-Thighs Crunches

(see page 78 for photo example)

**Muscle group targeted:** Rectus abdominus (stomach)

**SETUP/STARTING POSITION:** Lie down on your back with your knees bent and your feet flat on the floor. Your arms should be straight out in front of you with your palms resting on your thighs.

**MOVEMENT:**

**Positive Stage:** Keeping your chin tuched in, raise your shoulder blades off of the floor, moving your hands up your thighs.

**Negative Stage:** When you feel as though you cannot raise any higher, Slowly lower your shoulder blades and hands to the starting position.

> **Buddy's Tip:** Remember to exhale as you crunch and inhale as you lower your shoulders back down.

# BODY TONING: ADVANCED

## Program Guidelines

**Frequency:** 3 to 5 times per week

**Warm-up:** 5 minutes of light cardiovascular exercise: riding an exercise bike, walking on a treadmill, doing jumping jacks, jogging, or walking in place

**Estimated workout time per circuit:** 10 minutes, not including the warm-up and cool-down

**Repetitions (reps):** 18 per exercise

**Rep Speed:** Use a 1 count (say "one-Mississippi" in your head) during the positive stage of the movement and again during the negative stage.

**Cardio moves:** There are three cardio moves for this body-toning routine:

1. Jumping rope

2. Doing rock climbers: To perform rock climbers, position your body like a sprinter's at the start of a race. Then alternate moving your legs; while one leg is moving forward, the other leg is moving back. Perform this move for 30 seconds.

3. Doing plyometrics (feet together jumping side to side): Start this cardio move by placing two bands parallel on the floor a few inches by apart. Stand on one side of the bands with your feet hip-width apart. Jump over the bands from side to side for 30 seconds.

**Breathing:** Keep breathing during the exercises and cardio segments.

**Cool-down:** 5 minutes of light cardiovascular exercise: riding an exercise bike, walking on a treadmill, doing jumping jacks, jogging, or walking in place

## Making Progress

After completing one full circuit, see how you feel. If you can, try to complete another two circuits. The ultimate goal over time is to complete three consecutive full circuits of this advanced body-toning program.

## Exercise 1. Squat with Hands Up

**Muscle group targeted:** Quadriceps and gluteus maximus (thighs and buttocks)

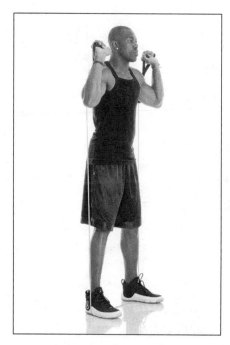

**SETUP/STARTING POSITION:** Stand on a band with your feet hip-width apart and pointing forward. Make sure that the length of the band from the outside of your shoe to the handle is the same on both sides. Bend down and grip a handle in each hand. With the bands behind your arms, raise the handles to shoulder height and rotate your palms so that they are facing forward. Keep your knees slightly bent and your chest up.

**MOVEMENT:**

**Negative Stage:** Lower your body until your thighs are parallel with the floor.

**Positive Stage:** Push from your heels and raise your body back to the starting position.

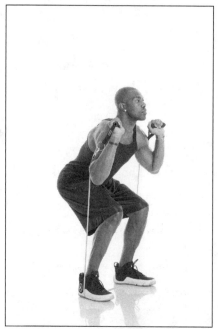

**Buddy's Tip** This is an incredible exercise for strengthening and shaping the entire leg. It will take some practice to master, so don't give up! Start the negative stage of the movement by sticking out your buttocks, similar to the motion required for sitting in a chair. Make sure that your knees are not pushing in toward each other or bowing out. If this is the case, decrease the resistance.

Perform one of the three specified cardio moves for 30 seconds.

# Exercise 2. Bent-over One-Arm Row

**Muscle group targeted:** Latisimus dorsi (middle and outer back)

**SETUP/STARTING POSITION:** Lay a band on the floor in front of you. Stand on the band with your left foot 12 inches from the right handle. Position your right leg back and lean forward. Grip the right handle with your right hand, keeping your upper arm perpendicular to the floor. Place your left hand on your left knee.

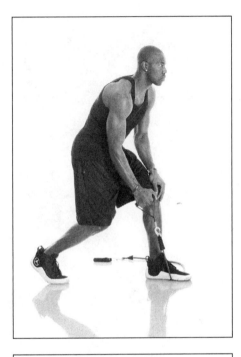

**MOVEMENT:**

**Positive Stage:** Pull the right handle up and back until it is next to your right hip.

**Negative Stage:** At a controlled speed, lower the handle forward and down until your right arm is perpendicular to the floor and back to the starting position.

Complete the desired number of reps and then switch sides.

**ALTERNATIVE RESISTANCE SOURCES:**
Dumbbells, standard-sized canned food

**Buddy's Tip** Create the pelvic tilt during this exercise by tightening your stomach muscles and pulling your buttocks forward and upward. To create the proper form while you are pulling, imagine that you are placing a coin in your back pocket. To help isolate your back muscles, keep a closed but loose grip on the handle.

Perform one of the three specified cardio moves for 30 seconds.

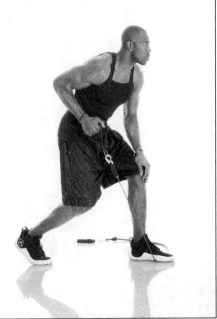

## Exercise 3. Lunge

**Muscle group targeted:** Quadriceps and gluteus maximus (thighs and buttocks)

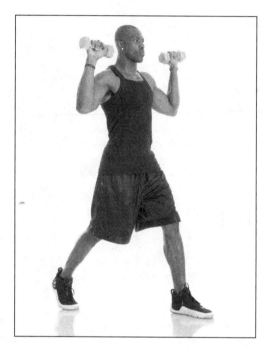

**SETUP/STARTING POSITION:** Grip a dumbbell in each hand and stand up straight with your left foot forward. Raise the dumbbells to shoulder height and rotate your palms so that they are facing forward. Your left knee should be slightly bent.

**MOVEMENT:**

**Negative Stage:** Keeping your chest up, lower your body until your left leg is parallel with the floor.

**Positive Stage:** Push from your heel and raise your body until your left leg is back at the starting position.

Complete the desired number of reps and then switch sides.

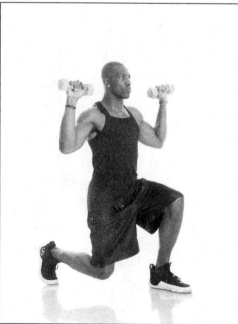

> **Buddy's Tip**  The knee of your front leg should not move forward during the exercise. The rule of thumb is that your front knee should be directly above the toes of your front foot.

Perform one of the three specified cardio moves for 30 seconds.

# Exercise 4. Standing One-Arm Triceps Extension

**Muscle group targeted:** Triceps (back of arms)

**SETUP/STARTING POSITION:** Stand up straight with your right foot just in front of your left. Step on the left end of a band with your right foot so that there is about 3½ feet of band between the outside of your right foot and a handle. With your right hand, grip the handle on the outside of your right foot and stand up straight. Keep the band behind your arm and raise the handle to the back of your neck. Position your arm so that your elbow is straight up. Put your left arm behind your back so that your palm is touching the band. Keep your knees slightly bent and your head straight.

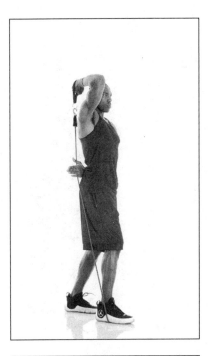

**MOVEMENT:**

**Positive Stage:** Push your hand straight up until your arm is almost totally extended.

**Negative Stage:** At a controlled speed, lower your hand to the starting position.

Complete the desired number of reps and then switch sides.

**ALTERNATIVE RESISTANCE SOURCE:** Dumbbells

> **Buddy's Tip** Create the pelvic tilt by tightening your stomach muscles and pulling your buttocks forward and upward. Be sure to keep your elbow up during the movement. If you are unable to do this, you can practice your form in front of a mirror or try decreasing the resistance.

Perform one of the three specified cardio moves for 30 seconds.

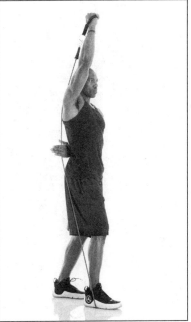

## Exercise 5. Hammer Curl

**Muscle group targeted:** Biceps (front of arms)

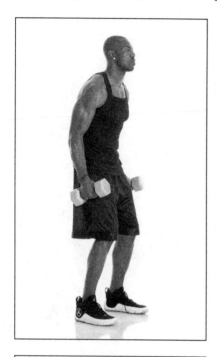

**SETUP/STARTING POSITION:** Grip a dumbbell in each hand and stand up straight with your feet hip-width apart. Keep your arms down at your sides with your palms resting on your outer thighs. Keep your knees slightly bent and your head straight.

**MOVEMENT:**

**Positive Stage:** Raise the dumbbells forward and up until they are at chest height.

**Negative Stage:** At a controlled speed, lower the weights until they are back at the starting position.

> **Buddy's Tip** Create the pelvic tilt by tightening your stomach muscles and pushing your buttocks forward and upward. Keep your elbows stationary at your sides. Do not move your elbows forward or back as you raise the dumbbells.

Perform one of the three specified cardio moves for 30 seconds.

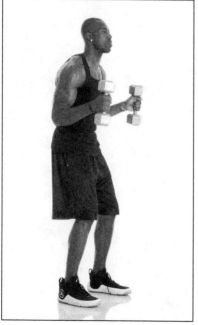

# Exercise 6. Standing Lateral Raise

**Muscle group targeted:** Medial deltoid (side shoulder)

**SETUP/STARTING POSITION:** Stand on a band with your feet hip-width apart. Make sure that the length of the band from the outside of your shoe to the handle is the same on both sides. Reach down and grip a handle in each hand. Stand up straight with your arms at your sides and your palms facing in toward each other. Keep your knees slightly bent.

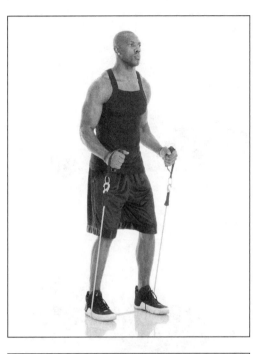

**MOVEMENT:**

**Positive Stage:** Raise your arms straight out to the sides until your elbows reach shoulder height.

**Negative Stage:** At a controlled speed, lower your arms to the starting position.

> **Buddy's Tip** Before you start the movement, create the pelvic tilt by tightening your stomach muscles and pulling your buttocks forward and upward. Keep your elbows higher than your hands as you raise your arms. A great trick to help you use proper form is to imagine that you are pouring milk out of cartons as you raise your arms.

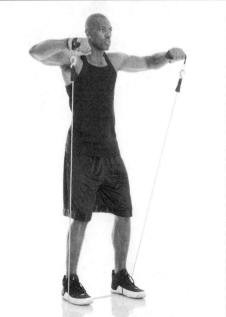

Perform one of the three specified cardio moves for 30 seconds.

## Exercise: 7. Resisted Push-up

**Muscle group targeted:** Pectoralis major (chest)

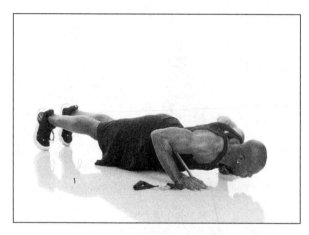

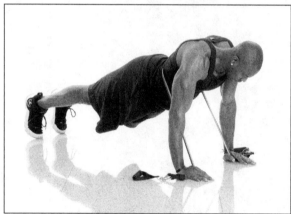

**SETUP/STARTING POSITION:** Wrap a band around your body so that it is around your back and the handles are in your hands. Lie facedown on the floor with your legs straight. Position your arms straight out to the sides with your hands directly under your elbows. Place your palms over the band on the floor so that it does not have any slack.

**MOVEMENT:**

**Positive Stage:** Keeping your head straight, push from your palms and raise your body off the floor until your arms are almost fully extended.

**Negative Stage:** At a controlled speed, lower your body to the starting position.

> **Buddy's Tip** Before you push up against the resistance for the first rep, make sure your pelvis is in the right position. To create the right position, tighten your stomach muscles and pull your buttocks down toward the floor and up toward your head. Do not let your midsection droop as you push your body off the floor. A side view should show your body straight as a board.

## Exercise 8. Superman Back Extension

**Muscle group targeted:** Erector spinae (lower back)

**SETUP/STARTING POSITION:** Lie facedown on the floor with your arms extended straight over your head and your legs straight. Keep your hands and feet a few inches more than shoulder-width apart. Place your palms flat on the floor.

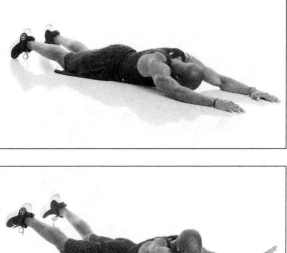

**MOVEMENT:**

**Positive Stage:** Raise your chest and thighs simultaneously 2 to 3 inches off the ground.

**Negative Stage:** At a controlled speed, lower your arms and legs to the starting position.

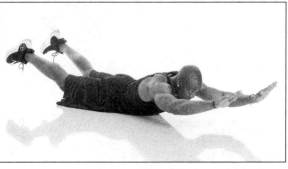

**Buddy's Tip** For those of you who need to strengthen your lower back, this is a supereffective and safe exercise. This exercise may take some time to master. As you raise your upper body off the ground, keep your head straight at the same level as your arms.

## Exercise 9. Folded-Arm Crunches

**Muscle group targeted:** Rectus abdominus (stomach)

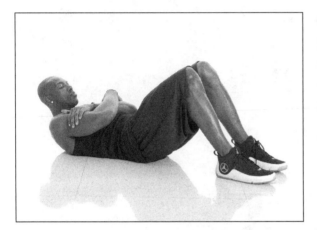

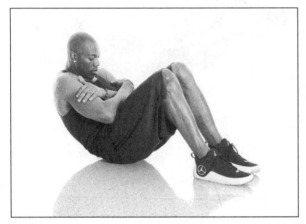

**SETUP/STARTING POSITION:** Lie on your back with your legs bent and your feet flat on the floor. Cross your arms over your chest so that your right hand is on your left shoulder and vice versa.

**MOVEMENT:**

**Positive Stage:** Keeping your chin tucked in, raise your shoulder blades off of the floor, moving your elbows toward your thighs.

**Negative Stage:** When you feel as though you cannot raise any higher, slowly lower your shoulder blades back to the starting position.

> **Buddy's Tip** Tighten your stomach muscles and pull your buttocks forward toward the ceiling and up toward your head. Remember to exhale as you crunch and inhale as you lower your shoulders back down.

## BUILDING MUSCLE

One of the best ways to build muscle is to tear it down, let it heal, and then tear it down again. After years of trial and error, a great number of elite athletes discovered a workout schedule that leaves the optimal amount of time between your workouts. The schedule splits up your training sessions so that you work each specific muscle group three times every two weeks.

The exercises below are performed at the advanced level; however, you can change the level to intermediate or beginner by adjusting the weight according to the suggestions below.

First, let's take a look at the general guidelines.

### General Information

Perform the exercises in the order specified. Complete the desired number of sets per exercise, and then move on to the next exercise.

### Workout 1

**Chest exercises:** Resisted Push-up with Legs Crossed (page 85), Standing One-Arm Chest Fly (page 81)

**Triceps exercises:** Standing Triceps Extension (page 97), Two-Arm Kickback (page 82)

**Biceps exercises:** Standing Biceps Curl (page 83), Seated Hammer Curl (page 95)

### Workout 2

**Back exercises:** Overhead Lat Pull (page 98), Seated Back Row (page 84), Good Morning (page 86)

**Shoulder exercises:** Front Shoulder Raise (page 87), Standing Lateral Raise (page 88), Shrugs (page 91), Standing Rear Shoulder Pull (page 92)

**Stomach exercises:** Alternating Slant Board Crunches (page 94), Resisted Crunch (page 89)

## Workout 3

**Leg exercises:** Seated Leg Extension (page 99), Leg Press (page 93), Lying Leg Curl (page 90), Seated Calf Extension (page 96)

## Program Guidelines

**Frequency:** Each muscle group is worked three times every two weeks, per the schedule below.

**Warm-up and cool-down:** 5 minutes of light cardiovascular exercise: riding an exercise bike, walking on a treadmill, light jogging, or walking in place

**Sets:** 3 per exercise

**Repetition (reps):** 8 to 10 per set

**Rep speed:** For this program use a 1 count (say "one-Mississippi" in your head) during the positive stage of the movement and again during the negative stage.

**Breathing:** Be sure to exhale during the positive stage of the movement.

Here is how to space out the workouts over a two-week period.

**Week 1**

| Monday | Tuesday | Wednesday | Thursday | Friday | Saturday | Sunday |
|--------|---------|-----------|----------|--------|----------|--------|
| Work out | Work out | Work out | Day off | Work out | Work out | Day off |
| 1 | 2 | 3 | | 1 | 2 | |

**Week 2**

| Monday | Tuesday | Wednesday | Thursday | Friday | Saturday | Sunday |
|--------|---------|-----------|----------|--------|----------|--------|
| Work out | Day off | Work out | Work out | Work out | Day off | Day off |
| 3 | | 1 | 2 | 3 | | |

# Exercise 1. Standing One-Arm Chest Fly

**Muscle group targeted:** Pectoralis major (chest)

**SETUP/STARTING POSITION:** Anchor a band at chest height and attach both ends to one handle (you can also hold two handles in one hand). Grip the handle with your right hand and turn your body so that your right shoulder is facing the anchor point. Position your right arm out to the side so that it is parallel with the floor with a slight bend. Rotate your hand so that your thumb is on top. Move your body far enough from the anchor point that there is a slight amount of tension on the band. Keep your left hand on your left hip and your knees slightly bent.

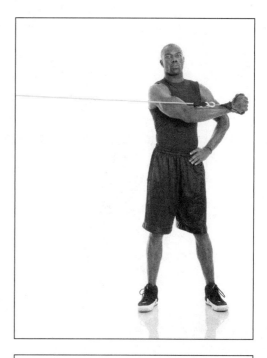

**MOVEMENT:**

**Positive Stage:** Pull the handle out and across your body until it is just past the center of your chest.

**Negative Stage:** At a controlled speed, return the handle to the starting position.

Complete the desired number of reps and then switch sides.

**ALTERNATIVE RESISTANCE SOURCE:** Gym cable machine

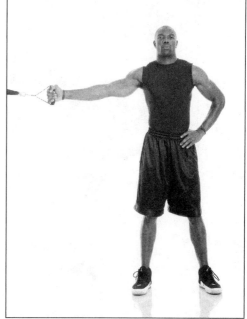

**Buddy's Tip** Adjust your stance to incorporate the pelvic tilt: tighten your stomach muscles and push your buttocks forward and upward. Do not bend your working arm too much as you pull the handle across your body. Try to imagine that your arm naturally has a slight bend and is fused that way. If you have trouble, try lowering the amount of resistance.

## Exercise 2. Two-Arm Kickback

**Muscle group targeted:** Triceps (back of arms)

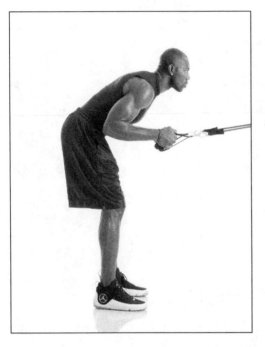

**SETUP/STARTING POSITION:** Anchor a band at stomach height and grip a handle in each hand. Face the anchor point and step back. Your distance from the anchor point should be far enough that there is a slight amount of tension on the band. Keep your waist slightly bent. Raise your upper arms until they are almost parallel with the floor and hold them tight to your body.

**MOVEMENT:**

**Positive Stage:** Keeping your elbows stationary, push the handles back until your arms are almost straight.

**Negative Stage:** At a controlled speed, return your arms to the starting position.

**ALTERNATIVE RESISTANCE SOURCE:** Dumbbells

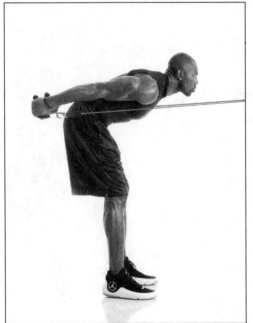

> **Buddy's Tip**  Create a strong center with the pelvic tilt: tighten your stomach and push your buttocks forward and upward. It is extremely important for your arms to stay tight to your body. Your elbows should not move up or down excessively as you push back.

# Exercise 3. Standing Biceps Curl

**Muscle group targeted:** Biceps (front of arms)

**SETUP/STARTING POSITION:** Stand on a band with your feet hip-width apart. Make sure that the length of the band from the outside of your shoes to the handles is the same on both sides. Grip a handle in each hand and stand up straight. Your arms should be perpendicular to the floor with your palms facing forward. Keep your knees slightly bent.

**MOVEMENT:**

**Positive Stage:** Keeping your elbows stationary at your sides, raise the handles until they are at chest height.

**Negative Stage:** At a controlled speed, lower the handles to the starting position.

**ALTERNATIVE RESISTANCE SOURCES:** Dumbbells, barbell

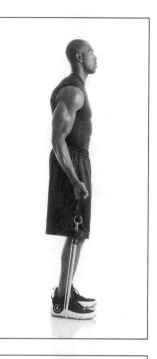

**Buddy's Tip** There are two very important tips that will help you properly isolate and work your biceps. The first is that your body must stay still; do not try to rock your body to raise the handles. One way to help stabilize your body is with, yep, you guessed it, the pelvic tilt: tighten your stomach and push your buttocks forward and upward. The second tip is that your elbows must stay in one place. Try not to move your elbows forward or backward as you raise the handles.

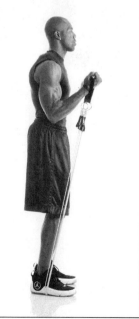

## Exercise 4. Seated Back Row

**Muscle group targeted:** Latissimus dorsi (middle and outer back)

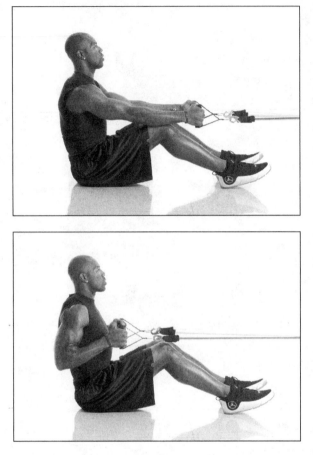

**SETUP/STARTING POSITION:** Anchor a band at knee height. Grip a handle in each hand and face the anchor point. Sit down with your knees bent and your heels on the floor. Move far enough away from the anchor point that there is a slight amount of tension on the band. Your arms should be straight out in front of you, parallel with the floor. Rotate your wrists so that your thumbs are on top.

**MOVEMENT:**

**Positive Stage:** Pull the handles back with your elbows down and your arms tight to your body.

**Negative Stage:** At a controlled speed, return the handles to the starting position.

**ALTERNATIVE RESISTANCE SOURCE:** Gym cable machine

> **Buddy's Tip** Do not grip the handles tightly, as this will cause you to start pulling with your biceps instead of your back. Keep your hands closed but loose around the handles.

# Exercise 5. Resisted Push-up with Legs Crossed

**Muscle Group Targeted:** Pectoralis major (chest)

**SETUP/STARTING POSITION:** Wrap a band around your body so that it is around your back and the handles are in your hands. Lie facedown on the floor with one leg crossed over the other. Position your arms straight out to the side with your hands directly under your elbows. Place your palms over the band on the floor so that it does not have any slack.

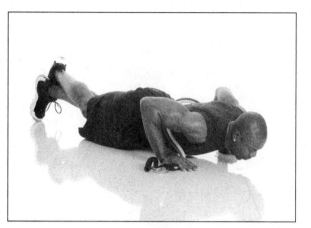

**MOVEMENT:**

**Positive Stage:** Keeping your head straight, push from your palms and raise your body off the floor until your arms are almost straight.

**Negative Stage:** At a controlled speed, lower your body to the starting position.

**ALTERNATIVE RESISTANCE SOURCES:** Bench with dumbbells or barbells

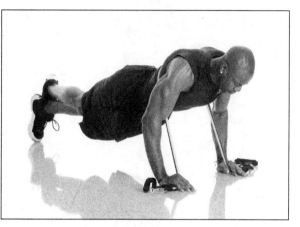

> **Buddy's Tip** Before you push up against the resistance for the first rep, make sure your pelvis is in the right position. To create the right position, tighten your stomach muscles and pull your buttocks down toward the floor and up toward your head. Do not let your midsection droop as you raise your body. A side view of your body should show your body straight as a board.

## Exercise 6. Good Morning

**Muscle group targeted:** Erector spinae (lower back)

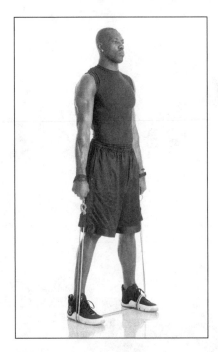

**SETUP/STARTING POSITION** Bend down and step on a band with your right foot so that there are 8 inches from the outside of your foot to the handle. Wrap the other end of the band around your left foot once. Make sure that the length of the band from the outside of your shoe to the handle is the same on both sides. Grip the handles and stand up straight. Your hands should be straight down with the palms of your hands resting on your outer thighs. Keep your knees slightly bent and shoulder-width apart.

**MOVEMENT:**

**Negative Stage:** At a controlled speed, bend from your waist and lower your upper body until your hands are touching the outside of your knees.

**Positive Stage:** Raise your upper body to the starting position.

**ALTERNATIVE RESISTANCE SOURCES:** Dumbbells, barbell

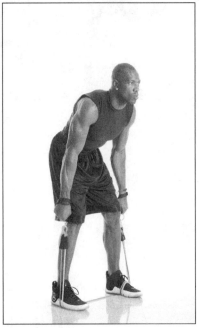

> **Buddy's Tip** Make sure you do not hyperextend your neck as you lower your body.

## Exercise 7. Front Shoulder Raise

**Muscle group targeted:** Anterior deltoid (front shoulder)

**SETUP/STARTING POSITION:** Stand on a band with your feet hip-width apart. Make sure that the length of the band from the outside of your shoe to the handle is the same on both sides. Grip a handle in each hand and stand up straight with your knees slightly bent. Your arms should be at your sides, tight to your body and almost fully extended. Rotate your hands so that your palms face your thighs.

**MOVEMENT:**

**Positive Stage:** Raise your arms until they are parallel with the floor.

**Negative Stage:** At a controlled speed, return your arms to the starting position.

**ALTERNATIVE RESISTANCE SOURCES:** Gym cable machine, dumbbells

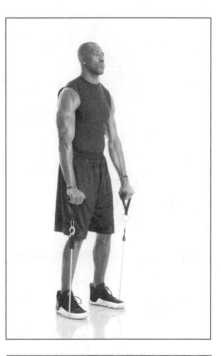

> **Buddy's Tip** As you are getting into your starting position, implement the pelvic tilt: tighten your stomach and pull your buttocks forward and upward. When you raise the handles, try not to bend your arms too much and keep your hands separated and shoulder-width apart.

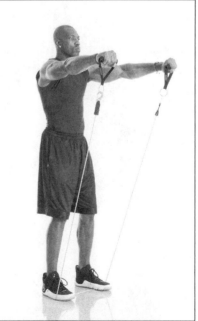

## Exercise 8. Standing Lateral Raise

**Muscle group targeted:** Medial deltoid (side shoulder)

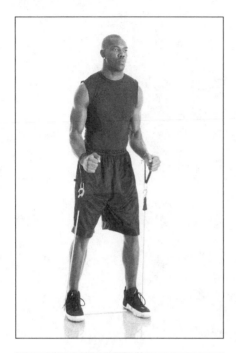

**SETUP/STARTING POSITION:** Stand with your feet hip-width apart on a band. Make sure that the length of the band from the outside of your shoe to the handle is the same on both sides. Reach down and grip a handle in each hand. Stand up straight with your arms at your sides and your palms facing in toward each other. Keep your knees slightly bent.

**MOVEMENT:**

**Positive Stage:** Raise your arms straight out to the side until your elbows reach shoulder height.

**Negative Stage:** At a controlled speed, lower your arms to the starting position.

**ALTERNATIVE RESISTANCE SOURCE:** Dumbbells

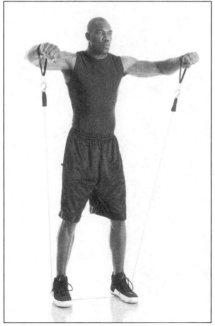

**Buddy's Tips** Before you start the movement, create the pelvic tilt by tightening your stomach muscles and pulling your buttocks forward and upward. Keep your elbows higher than your hands as you raise your arms. A great trick to help you use proper form is to imagine that you are pouring milk out of cartons as you raise your arms.

# Exercise 9. Resisted Crunch

**Muscle group targeted:** Rectus abdominus (stomach)

**SETUP/STARTING POSITION:** Anchor a band at floor level. Sit close to the anchor point with your back to the anchor point. Grip a handle in each hand and lie on your back with your knees bent and your feet flat on the floor. Keep your chin tucked in and your palms flat on the floor.

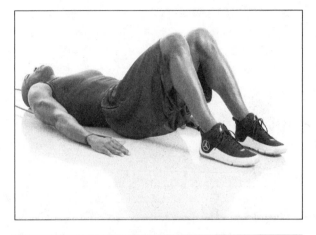

**MOVEMENT:**

**Positive Stage:** Push your hands toward your feet and raise your shoulders off the floor until you are unable to move your hands any farther.

**Negative Stage:** At a controlled speed, lower your shoulders to the starting position.

**ALTERNATIVE RESISTANCE SOURCE:** Gym cable machine

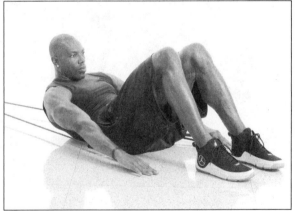

**Buddy's Tip** Adjust your starting position to incorporate the pelvic tilt by tightening your stomach muscles and moving your buttocks forward toward the ceiling and up toward your head. Remember to exhale as you crunch and inhale as you lower your shoulders back down.

## Exercise 10. Lying Leg Curl

**Muscle Group Targeted:** Hamstrings (back of legs)

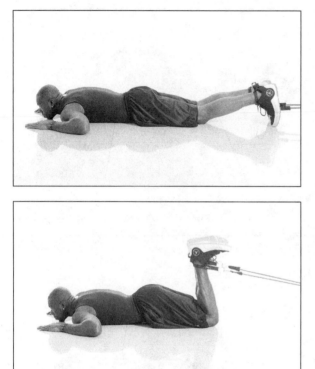

**SETUP/STARTING POSITION:** Anchor a band at floor level. Position your body with your back to the anchor point. Wrap the ankle straps around your ankles and lie chest down on the floor away from the anchor point. Your distance from the anchor point should be far enough that there is a slight amount of tension on the band. Place your palms flat on the floor to stabilize your body, and keep your head straight.

**MOVEMENT:**

**Positive Stage:** Keeping your knees and feet close together, bend your knees and move your heels toward your buttocks until your knees stop bending naturally.

**Negative Stage:** At a controlled speed, lower your legs to the starting position.

**ALTERNATIVE RESISTANCE SOURCE:** Gym leg-curl machine

**Buddy's Tip** Create the pelvic tilt by tightening your stomach muscles and moving your buttocks down into the floor and up toward your head. If you feel as though you are tightening your calves as you bend your legs, point your toes; this will disengage the calves and help isolate the hamstrings.

# Exercise 11. Shrugs

**Muscle group targeted:** Trapezius (upper shoulders)

**SETUP/STARTING POSITION:** Bend down and step on a band with your left foot so that there are 8 inches from the outside of your foot to the handle. Wrap the other end of the band around your right foot once. Make sure that the length of the band from the outside of your shoe to the handle is the same on both sides. Grip the handles and stand up with your knees slightly bent and your arms straight down by your sides.

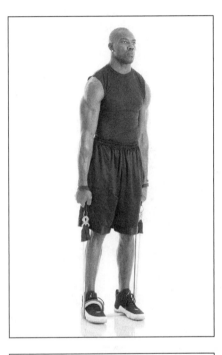

**MOVEMENT:**

**Positive Stage:** Raise your shoulders straight up until they stop naturally.

**Negative Stage:** At a controlled speed, lower your shoulders to the starting position.

**ALTERNATIVE RESISTANCE SOURCES:** Dumbbells, barbell

> **Buddy's Tip** As in most standing exercises, you will need to create a pelvic tilt to stabilize your body properly: tighten your stomach and pull your buttocks forward and upward. To generate the proper form for this exercise, attempt to touch your shoulders to your ears.

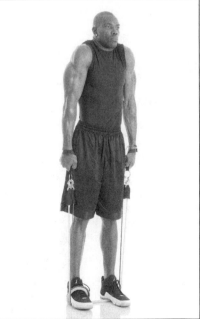

## Exercise 12. Standing Rear Shoulder Pull

**Muscle group targeted:** Posterior deltoid (rear shoulder)

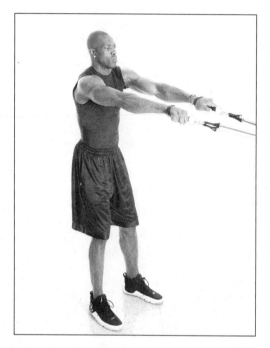

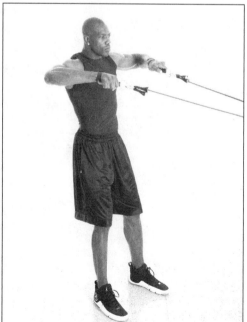

**SETUP/STARTING POSITION:** Anchor a band at chest height. Position your body so that you are facing the anchor point and grip a handle with each hand. Stand far enough away from the anchor point that there is a slight amount of tension on the band. Keep your arms straight out in front of you, parallel with the floor. Rotate your wrists so that your palms are facing toward the floor. Your feet and knees should be hip-width apart. Keep your knees slightly bent.

**MOVEMENT:**

**Positive Stage:** Pull the handles out and back until your arms stop naturally. At the end of the pull, your elbows should be bent at a 90-degree angle.

**Negative Stage:** At a controlled speed, move the handles back to the starting position.

**ALTERNATIVE RESISTANCE SOURCE:** Gym cable machine

> **Buddy's Tip** Create the pelvic tilt for this exercise by tightening your stomach muscles and pushing your buttocks forward and upward. As you pull back, lead with your elbows. Keep your head straight.

# Exercise 13. Leg Press

**Muscle group targeted:** Quadriceps (thighs)

**SETUP/STARTING POSITION:** Sit in a leg-press machine with the seat adjusted to a 45-degree angle. Place your feet on the pressing platform. Your knees and feet should be no more than hip-width apart, and your feet should be pointing straight ahead. Press the platform up and disengage the safety bars (typically by pushing them out to the side). Grip the side of the machine or handles (if available) to stabilize your body. This exercise is supereffective at strengthening the entire leg and is a key component in many elite training programs.

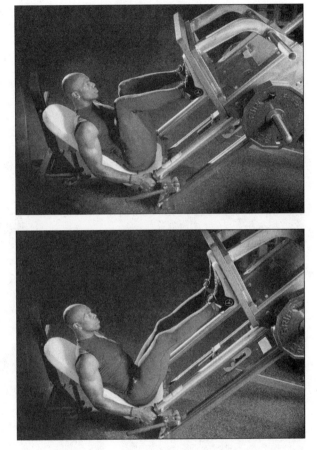

**MOVEMENT:**

**Negative Stage:** Lower the platform until your legs stop naturally.

**Positive Stage:** Pushing from your heels, raise the platform until you are back to the starting position.

When you are done with your set, reengage the safety bar.

**Buddy's Tip** You must incorporate the pelvic tilt during this exercise. To achieve this, tighten your stomach muscles and push your buttocks forward toward your feet and up toward the ceiling. Make sure that your knees do not move in or out as you are pushing, and do not lock them at the top. If you find it difficult to maintain the proper form, try reducing the amount of weight.

## Exercise 14. Alternating Slant Board Crunches

**Muscle group targeted:** Rectus abdominus (stomach)

**SETUP/STARTING POSITION:** Secure your feet and legs underneath the pads at the top of the slant board. Lower your body until your shoulders are about 18 inches from the back pad. Place your fingertips behind your head, keeping your elbows back.

**MOVEMENT:**

**Positive Stage:** Raise your chest up and touch your right elbow to your left knee.

**Negative Stage:** At a controlled speed, lower your shoulders to the starting position.

**Positive Stage:** Raise your chest up and touch your left elbow to your right knee.

**Negative Stage:** At a controlled speed, lower your shoulders back to the starting position.

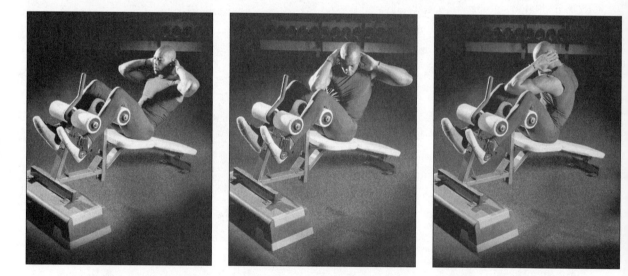

**Buddy's Tip**  To create the pelvic tilt for this exercise, tighten your stomach muscles and move your buttocks forward toward your feet and up toward the ceiling. Do not lock your hands behind your head and pull your neck to raise your chest. Be sure to exhale as you crunch.

## Exercise 15. Seated Hammer Curl

**Muscle group targeted:** Biceps (front of arms)

**SETUP/START POSITION:** Grip a dumbbell in each hand and sit on an upright bench. Place your feet flat on the floor or on a footrest, if available. Your knees and feet should be 6 inches apart. Sit up straight with your shoulders back and your arms hanging straight down. Rotate your wrists so that your palms are facing in toward each other.

**MOVEMENT:**

**Positive Stage:** Raise the dumbbells forward and up until they are at chest height.

**Negative Stage:** At a controlled speed, lower the weights to the starting position.

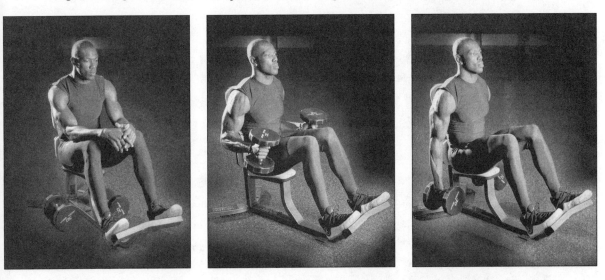

**Buddy's Tip** Incorporate the pelvic tilt into your seated position by tightening your stomach muscles and pushing your buttocks forward and upward. Isolate your biceps by keeping your upper body still; do not rock your body. Hold your elbows stationary at your sides. Try not to move them forward or backward as you raise the weight.

## Exercise 16. Seated Calf Extension

**Muscle group targeted:** Gastrocnemius and soleus (calf)

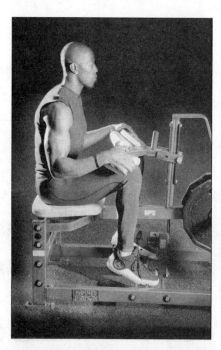

**SETUP/STARTING POSITION:** Sit on the calf-raise machine with the balls of your feet on the platform step and your knees directly under the knee pads. Your feet should be pointed straight ahead. Adjust the knee pads so that they are they are pressing down against your knees. Keep your chest up and your head straight. Raise your heels and disengage the safety bar (typically by pushing it out to the side), then lower your heels until they stop naturally.

**MOVEMENT:**

**Positive Stage:** Pushing from your big toe, raise your heels as high as you can before they stop naturally.

**Negative Stage:** At a controlled speed, lower your heels to the starting position.

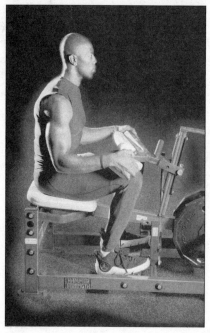

> **Buddy's Tip** Make sure that your body is in the proper position: when sitting upright on this machine, tighten your stomach and move your buttocks forward and upward.

## Exercise 17. Standing Triceps Extension

**Muscle group targeted:** Triceps (back of arm)

**SETUP/STARTING POSITION:** Stand up straight in front of a triceps cable machine and grip the rope or bar. Keep your knees slightly bent and your feet hip-width apart. Your elbows should be at your sides, and your upper arms should be perpendicular to the floor. Keep your shoulders down and a little forward.

**MOVEMENT:**

**Positive Stage:** Push the rope or handle straight down until your arms are almost fully extended.

**Negative Stage:** At a controlled speed, raise your hands to the starting position.

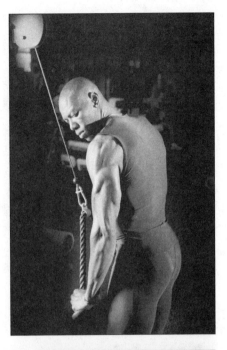

> **Buddy's Tips** Once again, definitely add the ever-so-important pelvic tilt to your stance: tighten your stomach and move your buttocks forward and up. Keep your elbows stationary at your sides. Try not to move them forward or backward as you push down.

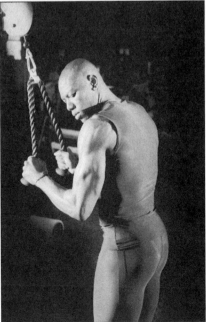

## Exercise 18. Overhead Lat Pull

**Muscle group targeted:** Latissimus dorsi (middle and outer back)

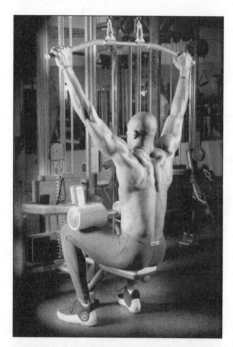

**SETUP/STARTING POSITION:** Before you pull the bar down, sit on the seat of the lat-pull machine and adjust the leg pads so that they are snug against your thighs. Set the weight and stand up. Grip the bar a few inches farther apart than shoulder-width. Pull the bar down and place your legs under the leg pads. Keep your shoulders down and your elbows back. Your upper body should lean back just a few inches.

**MOVEMENT:**

**Positive Stage:** Pull the bar down to the top of your chest.

**Negative Stage:** At a controlled speed, raise the bar to the starting position.

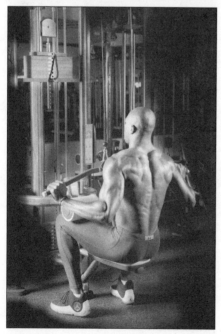

**Buddy's Tip** Once you have pulled the bar down and anchored your hand, add the pelvic tilt by tightening your stomach muscles and pushing your buttocks forward and upward. Keep a closed but loose grip around the bar; this will help isolate the back muscles.

# Exercise 19. Seated Leg Extension

**Muscle group targeted:** Quadriceps (thighs)

**SETUP/STARTING POSITION:** First, adjust the back-support pad so that when you sit in the leg-extension machine your knee is just past the end of the seat. Adjust the shin pad (if possible) so that the pad is just above ankle height. Position your legs so that your kneecaps are facing straight up to the ceiling. Grip the handholds (if available) or side of the seat to hold your buttocks down, and lean slightly forward.

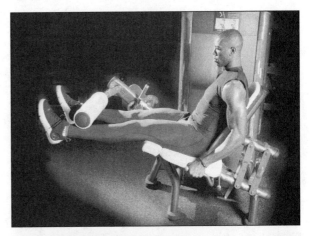

**MOVEMENT:**

**Positive Stage:** Pushing from your shins, raise the leg pad until your legs are almost fully extended.

**Negative Stage:** At a controlled speed, lower the leg pad to the starting position.

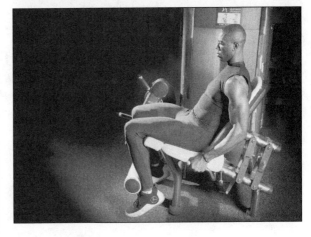

> **Buddy's Tip:** To achieve the pelvic tilt for this exercise, tighten your stomach muscles and push your buttocks forward and upward. If you feel that you are tightening your calf muscles during the exercise, point your toes. This will help take those muscles out of the movement.

# PART III

## The T.O. Diet

I'm going to show you how you can eat what you like and maintain a satisfying level of fitness. I will give you my own personal diet, during both the football season and the off-season. I will show you what my cheat sheet looks like and explain how I'm able to indulge in foods like sweets and still maintain my football form.

This section is broken down into three chapters, with two personal testimonies, and provides food lists, tips for healthful eating, and menu plans to follow while traveling or on the run. I'll even show you how to eat out and what to order when you're in a restaurant.

Because there are so many diet and fitness programs on the market today, it can be difficult to discern which one is right for you. I can help you unravel the mystery of diet and nutrition, focusing on how food plays a major role in any fitness plan and how you can develop a healthy lifestyle that can include all kinds of foods, even your favorites.

---

# 5

# Daily Discipline: What You Should Eat Every Day

**The key to any fitness and health program** is maintaining the right balance of diet, exercise, and rest. To maintain a peak level of performance, the ideal equation should be 60% diet/30% exercise/10% rest. And while you must be disciplined about your diet, discipline does not mean denial.

A disciplined diet will, of course, have a good balance of protein, carbohydrates, and fats and will include lean meats, fish, fruits, and vegetables. However, it is important to note that a disciplined diet does not mean that any particular food is off limits. The key to success is variation with moderation. By setting reasonable limits, you will be able to do what I do—indulge in all kinds of food, including pizza and even chocolate—and still maintain peak form.

The following plan can be used by anyone, of any age or gender.

## GENERAL BODY MAINTENANCE: MENU PLAN 1

If you want to ease your way into a more disciplined diet, this menu is for you.

### My Beverage of Choice

Water is pure liquid refreshment and accounts for a large percentage of what makes each of us human. The average 150-pound adult body contains 40 to 50 quarts of water. Almost two-thirds of our body weight is water weight:

**Blood is 80 percent water.**

**Muscles are 75 percent water.**

**The brain is 74 percent water.**

**Bone is 22 percent water.**

Because water makes up such a large portion of our body, and is essential for life, do yourself a favor: don't drink your calories. Raise a toast to a refreshing beverage that makes the most sense.

# Monday

### Breakfast:

**ADULTS**: Oatmeal

**TEENS**: Cold whole-grain cereal with 1% or skim milk

### Midmorning snack:

**ADULTS**: Banana or melon

**TEENS**: Granola bar and apple

### Lunch:

**ADULTS**: Tuna salad with 4 whole-grain crackers

**TEENS**: Turkey sandwich, protein shake, baked chips

### Midafternoon snack:

**ADULTS**: Low-fat yogurt

**TEENS**: Grapes

### Dinner:

**ADULTS/TEENS**:

Vegetable/chicken medley:

1–2 chicken breasts per person, grilled or baked, lightly seasoned or with lemon and olive oil

Assorted raw vegetables

1 whole-wheat roll or corn muffin

### Evening snack:

**ADULTS/TEENS**: Lightly salted popcorn

---

**Diet Myth 1**: *If I focus on sit-ups, I can get my waistline down.*

**T.O. Tool** Crunches work the abdominal muscles and can actually cause the muscle to expand. If there is a layer of fat atop the abdominal muscles, it may appear as if your stomach is protruding. To reduce your waistline, it is imperative to follow a well-balanced program of 60 percent diet, 30 percent exercise, and 10 percent rest.

## Tuesday

**Breakfast:**

**ADULTS/TEENS:** Oatmeal or whole-grain cereal with 1% or skim milk

**Midmorning snack:**

**ADULTS:** Sliced apples and mozzarella string cheese stick

**TEENS:** Banana or apple

**Lunch:**

**ADULTS:** Protein shake and mixed green salad

**TEENS:** Tuna sandwich, protein shake, baked chips

**Midafternoon snack:**

**ADULTS:** Low-fat yogurt

**TEENS:** Apple or low-fat yogurt

**Dinner:**

**ADULTS/TEENS:**
Roast beef stew:
Lightly seasoned roast beef, new potatoes, carrots, peas, and celery

1 biscuit, 1 piece of corn bread, or 1 whole-wheat roll

You can substitute lamb or lean pork roast for roast beef

**Evening snack:**

**ADULTS/TEENS:** A single serving of low-fat or sugar-free pastry, cookies, cake, or prepared desserts.

---

**Diet Myth 2:** *I must never eat after seven — or eight. Definitely not after nine!*

**T.O. Tool**  The only time you shouldn't eat after eight is if you're going to bed at nine. Our bodies are designed to be fed light, sensible meals every three to four hours. Without food every few hours, the body moves into starvation mode and begins to burn muscle and store fat. Not eating after seven or eight, if you're going to bed three or four hours later, may actually cause you to *gain* weight. For best results, eat until approximately ninety minutes before you retire for the night.

# Wednesday

### Breakfast:

**ADULTS**: Oatmeal and whole-grain English muffin

**TEENS**: Cream of Wheat, toast with peanut butter

### Midmorning snack:

**ADULTS**: Sliced pears with a serving of fat-free Cool Whip

**TEENS**: Pear or apple

### Lunch:

**ADULTS**: Chicken or tuna salad sandwich and baked chips

**TEENS**: Chicken or tuna salad sandwich, protein shake, cookies

### Midafternoon snack:

**ADULTS**: Raisins and fruit cup

**TEENS**: Nuts (no more than 20)

### Dinner:

**ADULTS/TEENS**: Whole-wheat spaghetti with meat sauce made with lean ground turkey. Large salad (lettuce, tomato, carrots, and any other raw vegetables you desire). 1 slice whole-wheat garlic toast or 1 whole-wheat roll

### Evening snack:

**ADULTS/TEENS**: Ice cream and 1 or 2 cookies (low-fat or sugar-free preferred)

---

**Diet Myth 3:** *Muscle can turn into fat!*

**T.O. Tool**  Can wood turn into steel? No! Muscle and fat are completely different cells that can never be converted into each other. Muscle will never become fat; fat will never become muscle. If you stop working out, your muscles will become smaller—and if you continue on the same diet, without exercising, your fat cells will expand. That often gives the appearance of muscle becoming fat, but that is not the case.

## Thursday

Breakfast:

**ADULTS**: Oatmeal or whole-grain cereal with 1% or skim milk

**TEENS**: Oatmeal or whole-grain cereal with 1% or skim milk

Midmorning snack:

**ADULTS**: Apple slices and low-fat string cheese stick

**TEENS**: Bananas and raisins

Lunch:

**ADULTS**: Baked chicken with a small salad

**TEENS**: Tuna salad sandwich, protein shake, snack-size package of baked chips

Midafternoon snack:

**ADULTS**: Low-fat yogurt

**TEENS**: Granola bar or raisins

Dinner:

**LEFTOVER NIGHT**: Anything you have left over from the week

Evening snack:

**ADULTS/TEENS**: Nuts

---

**Diet Myth 4:** *I'll just run it off.*

**T.O. Tool**  Years ago running was the solution for everything; however, studies show that walking (preferably up- and downhill) actually does more for your body than running will. For permanent weight loss, the focus has to be on altering your diet and switching to smaller meals eaten three to four hours apart.

# Friday

### Breakfast:

**ADULTS**: Cereal (any kind)

**TEENS**: Cereal (any kind)

### Midmorning snack:

**ADULTS**: Low-fat yogurt and string cheese stick

**TEENS**: Apple or orange

### Lunch:

**ADULTS**: Protein shake and salad

**TEENS**: Turkey sandwich and baked chips

### Midafternoon snack:

**ADULTS**: Fruit cup

**TEENS**: Raisins and nuts

### Dinner:

**ADULTS/TEENS**:
Salmon and noodles:
Grilled or baked salmon over noodles
dressed with light butter
Mixed green salad

### Evening snack:

**ADULTS/TEENS**: Lightly salted popcorn

---

**Diet Myth 5:** *There are no good carbs.*

**T.O. Tool**  The truth is that carbohydrates are like gasoline. The body needs easily accessed fuel—carbs—to run efficiently. There are no bad carbs. Some, like whole-grain bread and pasta, brown rice, and fruits and vegetables, are better than others. But all carbohydrates can be part of a healthy diet. The key to eating carbs is choosing quality and making smart decisions about the time of day you "fuel up." There's no need to eat a serving of pasta before bedtime. Common sense in planning will go a long way.

On the weekend, feel free to expand a bit on your of food choices, remembering to eat every three to four hours. Moderation is the key!

## Saturday

| | |
|---|---|
| **BREAKFAST**: Eggs served any way, turkey bacon, whole-wheat toast or whole-wheat waffle with light syrup or fresh fruit topping | **MIDMORNING SNACK**: Any fruit |
| **LUNCH**: Soup and any lean meat sandwich on whole-grain bread | **MIDAFTERNOON SNACK**: Low-fat or sugar-free cookies |
| **DINNER**: Pizza (veggie or limited to one meat topping and light cheese) with mixed green salad | **EVENING SNACK**: Ice cream or any other dessert (low-fat, sugar-free) |

---

**Diet Myth 6**: *Chicken and fish are best; never eat red meat!*

**T.O. Tool** Eaten in moderation, red meat is an important part of any healthy regimen. Red meat is necessary for building red blood cells, as well as strengthening your immune system. Lean meat, eaten twice a week, provides the body with essential nutrients such as protein, iron, zinc, and Vitamin B12. And contrary to popular belief, lean red meat is not a major source of cholesterol or fat.

## Sunday

**BREAKFAST**: Cream of Wheat, eggs, whole-grain toast

**MIDMORNING SNACK**: Fruit cup

**LUNCH**: Chicken chili, lettuce-and-tomato salad, whole-grain crackers

**MIDAFTERNOON SNACK**: Low-fat yogurt or raisins

**DINNER**: Baked chicken, lightly seasoned, with asparagus or broccoli cuts, or leftovers from any of the week's meals

**EVENING SNACK**: Dessert of your choice (low-fat or sugar-free)

---

**Diet Myth 7**: *The best way to lose weight is to skip a couple of meals.*

**T.O. Tool**  There is no doubt that if you skip a few meals, you will lose weight. What you'll also lose, however, is muscle. You may appear slimmer, but you will actually be "fatter" because your body is preserving fat while it burns muscle. Stick to the game plan and refuel your body every few hours. That's the best way to win!

Remember that you are what you eat and incorporate a variety of foods into your meal plans.

Processed food, such as frozen dinners, can be detrimental to your diet. While frozen diet meals may be low in calories, many are high in sodium, preservatives, and hidden fat. Eat as much fresh and natural food as possible.

## MODERATION IS THE KEY!

My food plan is not a diet; it's more a lifestyle decision to change your thoughts and habits. Diets are restrictive and difficult to stick to because of their nature. But with moderation, no food is off limits. Think about that: no denial, little temptation—a winning formula to achieving your goals!

---

**T.O. TESTIMONY:** *911 Emergency*

---

There are a lot of moments that will forever remain in the center of my mind. I remember the day I made it into the league and played in my first game. I remember my very first touchdown and having the courage to do my first touchdown dance. I remember my first day as a free agent, wondering what was ahead and where I'd end up. I remember my first on-field feud with an opposing team player. I remember hearing my first cheer and the first time I was booed. I remember how it felt to be the hot new thing and know how it feels to be a veteran player striving to stay relevant in the one game that I love.

Yet of all of those football memories, the one that stands out most clearly in my mind is September 28, 2006.

On September 26, I went to practice just as on any other day. I ran a few routes, rehabbed my injured hand, sat in meetings, watched game film, ate, and went home. I was in-season, so my training and diet routine remained the same, but I was off balance, primarily because there was a lot going on in my life.

On my mind was the drama of a failing relationship, as well as pressure from the media to perform at maximum level without doing anything remotely related to my "past personality." I was also trying to find my rhythm with a new team, new head coach, and new quarterback, all the while adjusting to life in a brand-new city.

Then there was my hand injury and the fact that, although I was a veteran player in the league, I was a rookie on this team. Not to mention that there were high expectations for my performance as a key player. Although the ink on my new contract was dry, I was still a stranger to Dallas.

On September 28th, I was sitting in a fog, trying to recall all that had happened while not believing everything that was being said and written about me. How did I go from trying to numb the pain I was feeling in my hand to hearing that I had attempted suicide? And those rumors were allegedly supported by police documents.

To this day, it's still unclear. What I can honestly say is that I was not trying to die. Regardless of the pressure, I had so much to live for.

I've never gone on record to say what went wrong the night of September 26, 2006. When asked if I was trying to kill myself, I can answer with confidence: No!

So what was the truth?

If living healthy and fully starts with the mind, mentally and emotionally on September 26, I was overwhelmed.

Even so, I continued to push my body. I maintained my disciplined workout routine because I was determined to be the best. I kept going because I wanted to believe that I had balance in my life, even though that wasn't true. I needed a rest—from everything and everybody.

Rest doesn't mean stop. Rest means rest! Really Establish "Still" Time.

There is a verse in scripture that I love that says, "Be still and know that I am God."

This was the verse that saved me then and helps me stay sane now, because I have defined what "rest" means *to* me and *for* me. Resting your mind and being still to the worries of this world is as essential to the body as breath. Stillness allows room for restoration, repair, and respect.

I respect the events of September 26, 2006, even with all the cruelness, mockery, and speculation that followed, because two days later on September 28, when the dust had barely settled, I found the meaning of rest. With every minute, hour, day, month, and year that passes, I learn that no matter what I face each day, no matter what ups or downs occur in- and off-season, I need to establish still time with myself; time to rejuvenate my mind, my body, and my spirit.

## THE DANGER OF DIETS

In order for you to have a healthful diet, everything negative around you must die. I love the word "diet" but not for normal reasons. I like to use the word "DIE-t" as a motivator and a symbol of what has to die in order for something else to live.

If I need to shed 5 pounds, run a 4.4, or rehab an injury quickly, I assess what has to die in order for me to do that. What I've learned from the night of September 26, 2006, was that if certain parts of my life are out of sorts—my relationships, my finances, my body, my emotions—I have to deal with those challenges by making clear and concise decisions on how to deal with them, establishing a clear timeline for completing those goals, and then proceeding with my plan of action.

I look at most people who go on diets, and at the end of eight to twelve weeks, they may be a tad smaller, but in two weeks or two months they are often back to the weight they were when they started. A diet has to provide a balance of food, fitness, and emotional stability. There is nothing worse than being emotionally stressed out while trying to accomplish the goal of becoming more physically fit.

After thirteen years in the league and having my share of turbulent and somewhat self-destructive seasons, I've discovered that the following things don't mix well when dieting:

1. Pills to remove pain in the midst of emotional pressure. (Take it from me: if you're not focused solely on the healing process when taking prescribed medicine, even if the dosage is correct, you are still vulnerable to error.)

2. Distress. I hate to hear about women who starve themselves for weeks in order to get into a dress at the last minute. Buy a bigger size or just don't go. Those kinds of diets never work. The results are temporary, and the stress they create for the body will surface later. You have only one body in this life—it is your responsibility to take care of it.

3. Hype. The only way to get into shape is to make a decision to do the work. That's why I decided to write a fitness book. People have asked me for years

what I do in order to maintain my body. My answer is and has always been the same: I made the decision, discovered a routine that worked, and then was willing to do (and actually did) the work necessary to achieve the results I wanted.

The reason this is so challenging for many people and the reason there is a greater failure rate than success rate with fitness programs is that people try too hard to conform to some type of one-size-fits-all guideline. Listen to me: find the thing (Pilates, gym, your home, DVDs, going to the park with the kids, football, basketball, tennis, golf, walking on the beach, running around the corner) that works best for you and do it.

The minute you try to conform to someone else's goals and don't get the results you want, you'll be left feeling as though you failed. You haven't failed; you just have to find a system that works for *you*.

Throughout the years, I've prided myself at taking bits and pieces from other players' games and making what I've learned from them my own. Jerry taught me a lot about speed and coordination. Shaq taught me a lot about strength. M.J. taught me about dedication. And my mom and grandmother taught me how to survive.

As far as workouts are concerned, I've watched and done it all. There are some exercises I really like and some I don't enjoy so much. I know which supplements, meals, and diet plans work for me and which, no matter how much they're hyped, don't work at all.

With the exercises and meal plans I've included in this book, there is something for everyone. Instead of dieting, prepare yourself to desert your past way of thinking and welcome the new you that you're destined to be.

# 6

# May I Have Some Chocolate, Please?

**This may come as a surprise,** but the short answer is yes! A few handfuls of M&M's or a small Snickers bar will not destroy your program.

In fact, chocolate and many other snacks can play an important role in your weight loss/maintenance program. Eating between meals not only can satisfy your cravings for chocolate or other sweets, it also helps maintain your metabolic level, helping you burn more calories throughout the day.

Though an occasional piece of chocolate is fine, when planning snacks, fruits and vegetables are best. The composition of these foods—water, vitamins, proteins, carbo-hydrates—makes the body work harder to digest them. Fruits and vegetables, with their natural enzymes, take longer to digest. Though all fruits and vegetables are good, the following guidelines can help you plan your program.

**Morning snack:** The key to this snack is to provide the body with energy. A bowl of strawberries is a satisfying sweet treat. Strawberries provide fuel, keeping your energy high and your brain working as your body moves toward the afternoon. (For an extra treat, serve with a little bit of fat-free Cool Whip.)

**Afternoon snack:** An apple in the middle of the day is an optimal fat-burning food. Apples, which are a wonderful combination of water and vitamins, hold water in the mus-cles and keep the body hydrated, which is crucial since our bodies are 78 percent water.

**Evening snack:** The evening snack can be a wonderful opportunity to burn a bit more fat before retiring for the night. A serving of raw carrots, for example, contains one hundred calories but burns two hundred calories during digestion. You're burning fat while you eat.

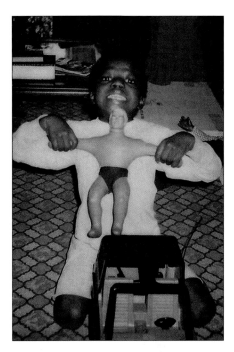

The Stretch Man was number one on Terrell's
Christmas list when he was six years old.
Even then he knew he wanted his body
to be able to do extraordinary things.

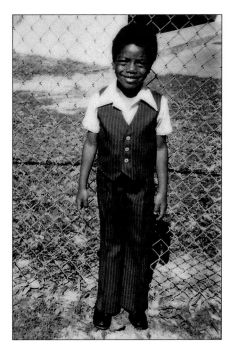

A bright and sunny day after church. Terrell's
mom made sure that her kids always looked
nice by making all of their clothes.

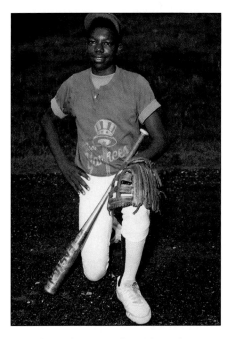

Terrell's mother describes his early teens
as his "odd years." His body was changing
rapidly, and sports became his only outlet.

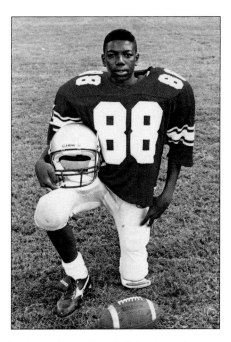

Benjamin Russell High School, sophomore
year: the wide receiver, age fifteen.

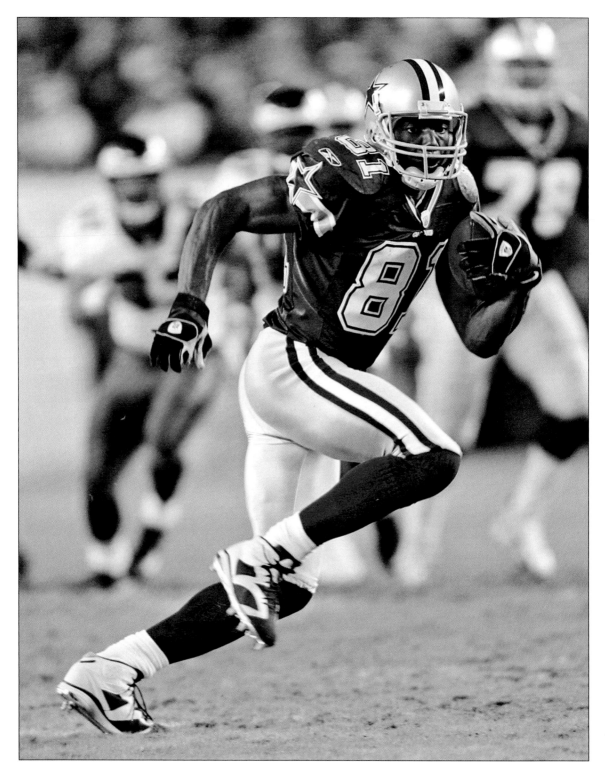

T.O. in motion.

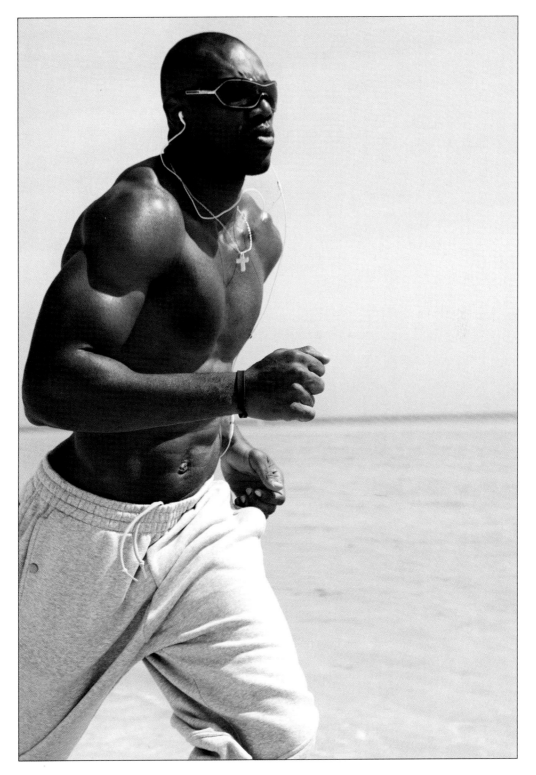

Running on the beach is a great way to clear your mind plus get some cardio.

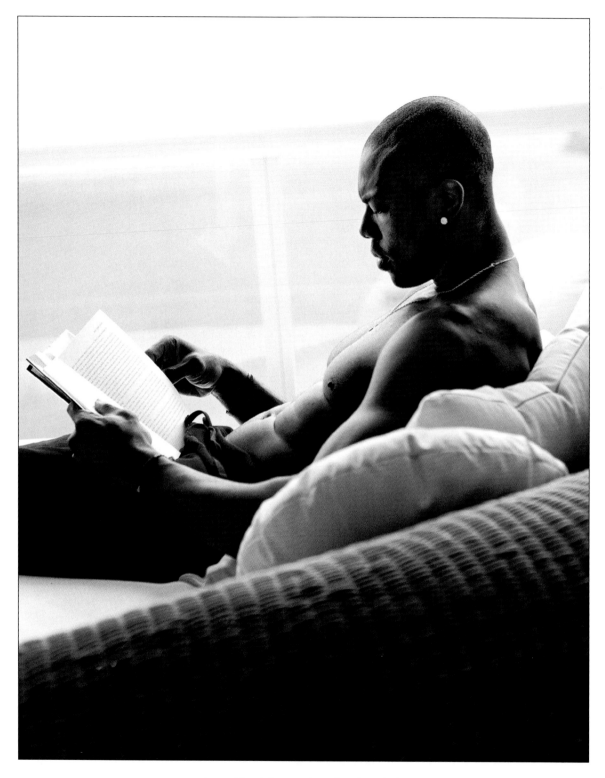

A good book is a workout for the mind.

I taught Andy Roddick
everything he knows.

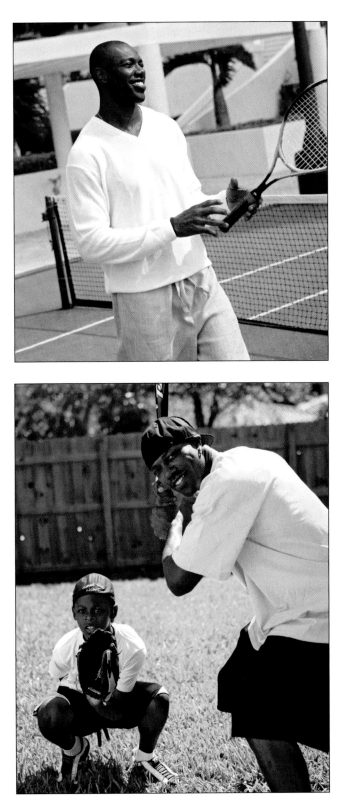

This one's going out of the park.

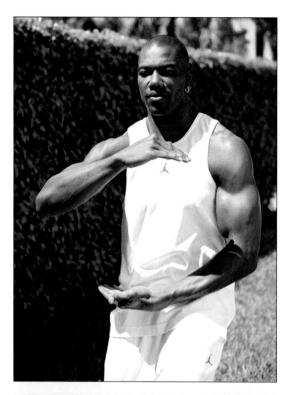

Tai chi helps balance
and flexibility.

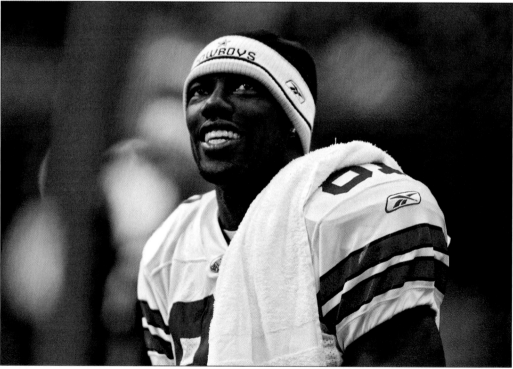

Who said winning wasn't everything!

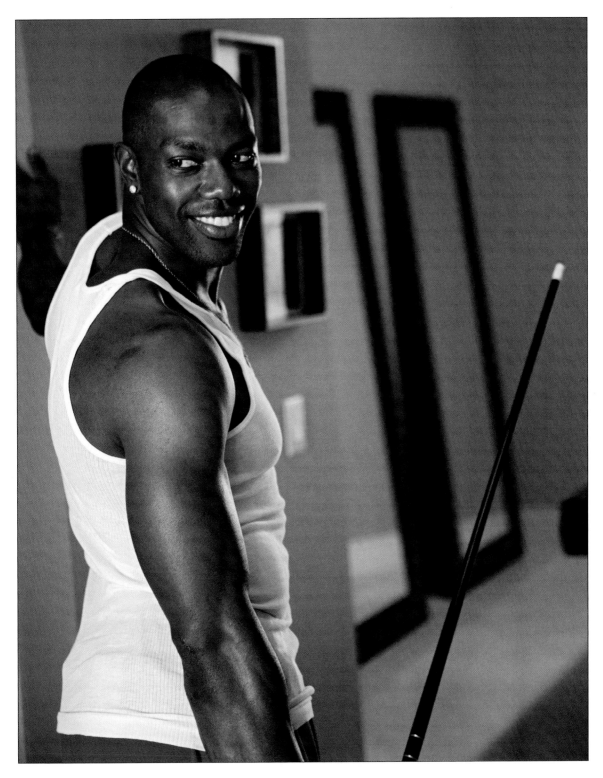

Do I *look* worried?

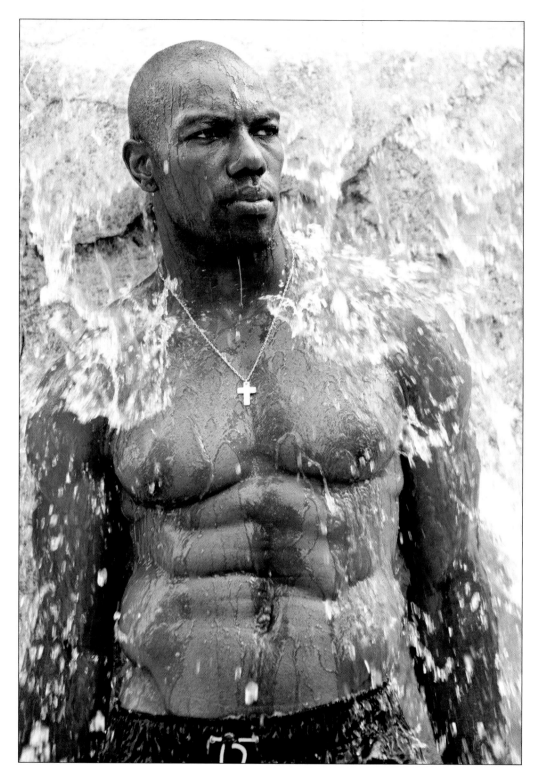

A little sumthin', sumthin'.

The man makes the suit.

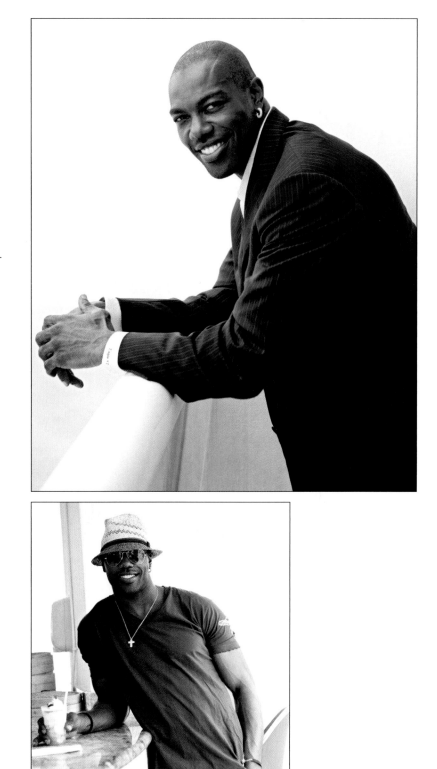

I Loves Me Some . . .

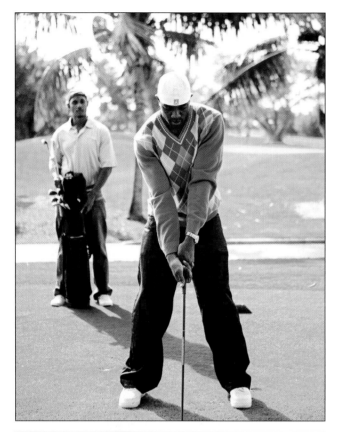

Watch out, Tiger!

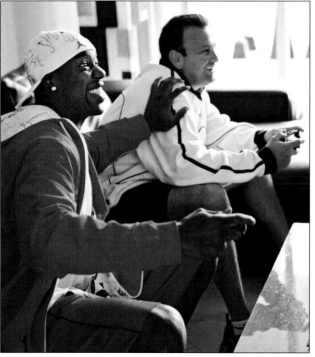

Hanging with my friend and
agent Drew Rosenhaus.

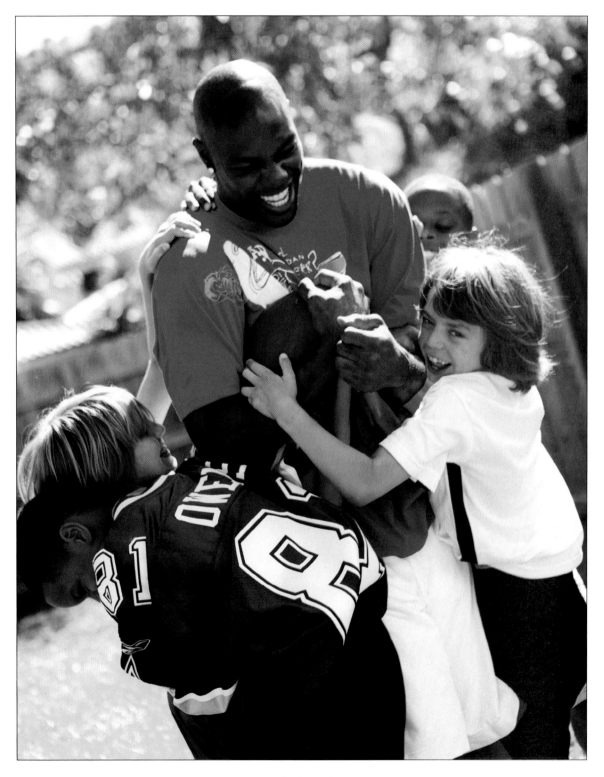

I'm still a kid at heart.

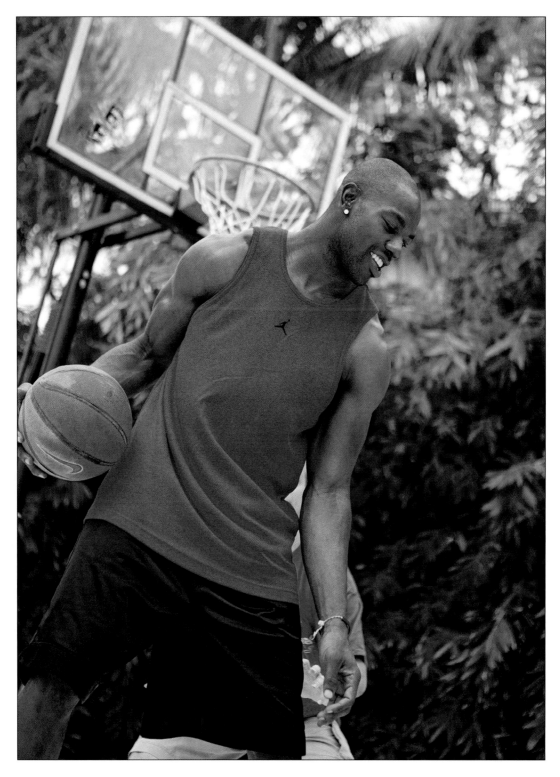

Basketball was always my first love.

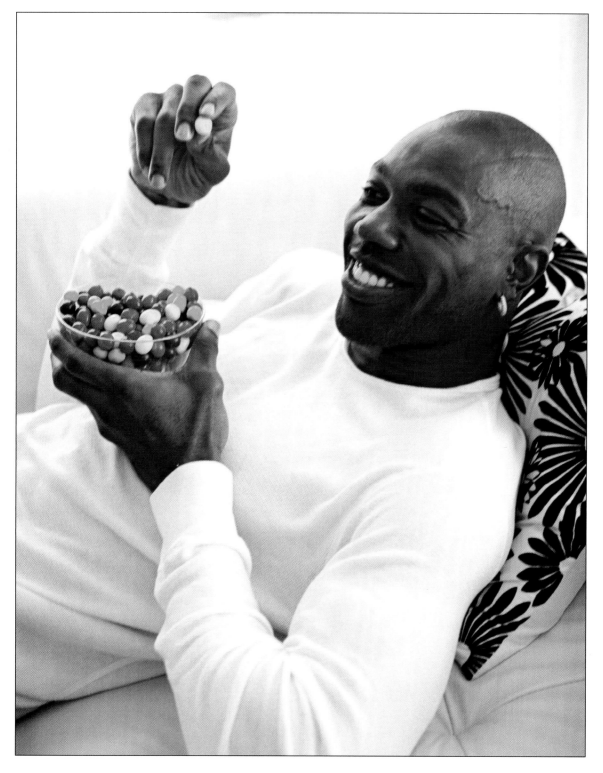

You can splurge a little with the proper balance.

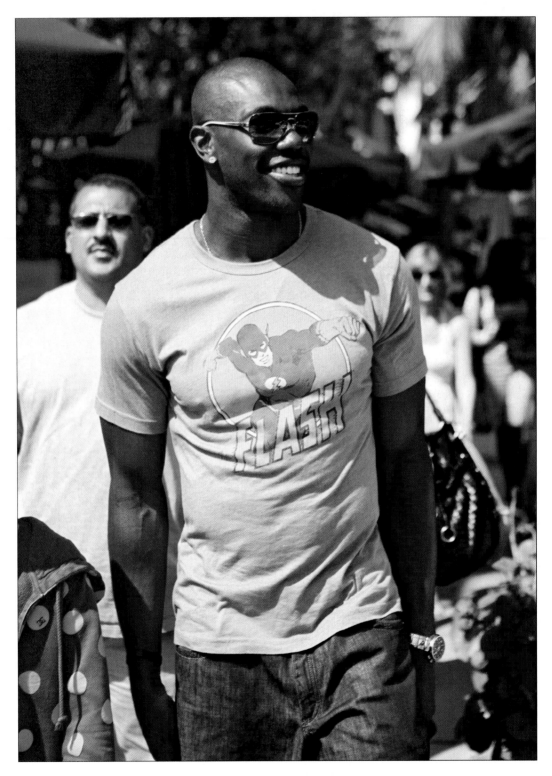

The T-shirt says it all.

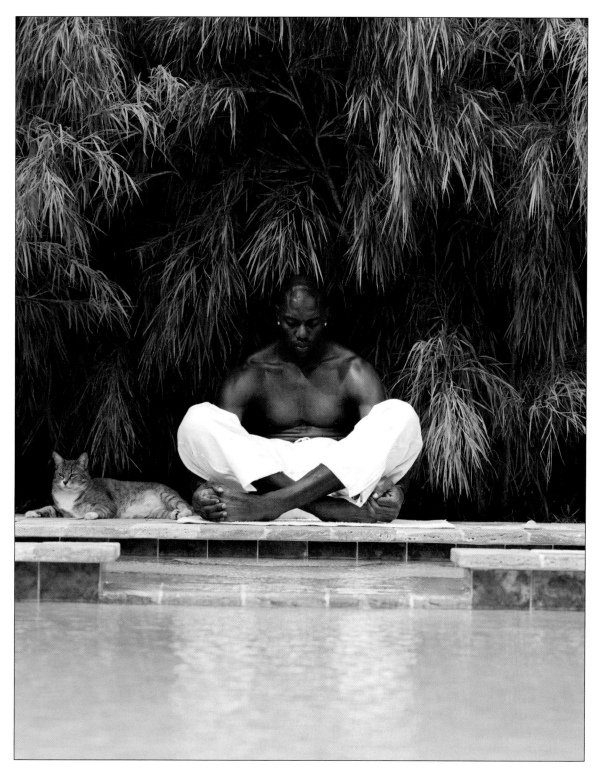

Achieving the mind, body, and spirit connection brings real power.

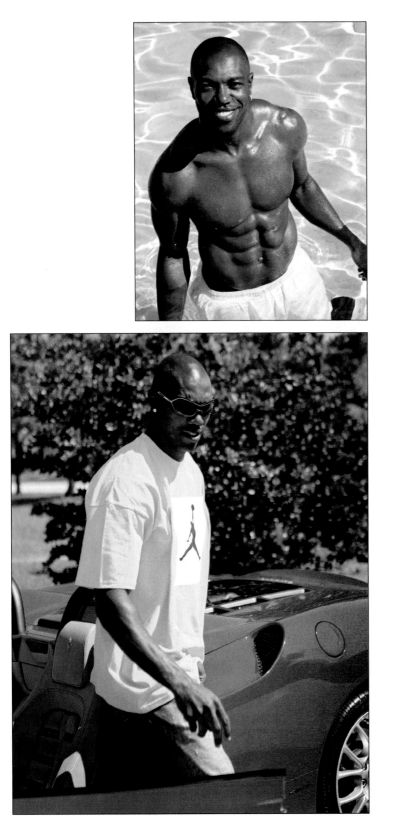

Refreshing.

Ferrari, the only thing
faster than me.

## CAKES, COOKIES, AND CANDY TOO!

As I've said before, nothing is off limits. But for optimal fitness, remember that the more natural the food, the better.

When preparing your own snacks and desserts, use all-natural products. When purchasing ready-to-eat products, look for the following:

### Cakes, Cookies, Pies, Coffee, Desserts

Stay away from products that contain white flour, fructose corn syrup, and simple sugars. Eating a processed food high in simple sugar, after an initial energy surge will leave you tired and dragging. This is an example of empty calories that do nothing for you.

### Ice cream, Candy, Puddings, Gum

Look for products that are low in sugar or sugar-free and low in fat.

### Syrups, Sweeteners, Natural Sugars

Again, natural products are best: honey, pure maple syrup, and, of course, fruit.

When thinking about any kind of dessert or snack, always consider timing. When is the best time to eat dessert? The earlier in the day, the better. Eat your last dessert or sweet snack at least two hours before you retire.

## ONE LITTLE DRINK CAN'T HURT A THING, RIGHT?

Even alcohol can be part of a healthy fitness program. There are some facts, however, that are important to consider:

- Alcohol breaks down into sugar.

- Alcohol inhibits the liver from breaking down fats.

- Two ounces or less of alcohol daily have been shown to reduce the risk of heart disease by 50 percent.

- On the other hand, *more* than two ounces daily can double your risk of heart disease and each one-ounce drink of alcohol stays with you—one to two pounds of water can remain in your body for two to three days!

To control the effects of alcohol consumption on your diet, consider the following:

- Vodka (with orange juice or lime) is low in sugar.

- Whiskey (with diet cola) is low in sugar.

- Scotch (with water) is low in sugar.

As with desserts, the keys to adding alcohol to your healthy diet are common sense and moderation.

## THE TRUTH ABOUT CALORIES

Counting calories has long been the mantra of American dieters. There is some validity to that; the equation, broken down into its simplest form, is this: calories in minus calories out equal the amount of weight lost or gained. However, counting calories is not enough.

For maximum fitness, the *quality* of calories you take in is more important than the *quantity*. Many foods are composed of empty calories—sodas, fried snacks, desserts made with refined sugar and white flour. They contain little nutritional value and may also be high in fat. Beware of these items, because they fill you with calories but provide little to your well-being and your body.

### T.O. TESTIMONY: *Getcha Grub On*

The notion that I work out for eight hours a day, seven days a week, eating only lean meat and vegetables, and that I sleep in a hyperbaric chamber every night is ridiculous. I *will* say that I've become very disciplined in how I treat my body, including what I put into it and what I allow to happen to it.

It's also ridiculous to think that just because I'm 6 foot 3 and weigh 200-plus pounds that I need to eat like a horse. On any given day, I average four to six small meals, including snacks. My portions are generally no larger than my hand; the size of my stomach is about the size of my fist, ensuring that I don't stuff myself.

Having grown up in the South, I'm accustomed to eating grits, greens, fatty meats smothered in God knows what, fried everything, including tomatoes, and loads of cakes, pies, cobblers, and cookies.

Just because that is what I grew up eating doesn't mean that's how I have to eat every day.

The flip side of the coin is that just because you grew up on fast food, it doesn't mean that they need to know you by your first name at your local fast-food joint.

I am no exception to the rule when it comes to wanting to getcha grub on. I like food, and I especially like good food with lots of flavor. But instead of knocking people over in the Thanksgiving line at Mom's house, I eat smart by taking smaller portions: I reach for one small piece of red velvet cake instead of two.

Food isn't about denial, it's about dosage—the amount you take in. Just because you can cook or even eat as if you're feeding an entire football team doesn't mean you have to. Take it easy, slow down, and relax; the food won't go anywhere. Once you monitor your portions, go ahead, getcha grub on.

# 7

# Let's Get Serious! The T.O. Diet Exposed

**For the first time,** I'm sharing my diet plans—programs that I follow both in-season and out. You will see two sides: my very rigid in-season plan, which allows me to operate at peak performance, and my off-season regimen, which allows me to indulge in anything I want and still maintain my football form. In this section, there are no rookies allowed. This isn't for the amateur, but by following this meal plan, you'll be in tiptop T.O. shape in no time.

## IN-SEASON

It's my job to keep my body in the best shape possible so that I can perform at an All-Star level. The following in-season plan provides my body with the best fuel possible. I eat the same meals every day, treating my body like a Ferrari, filling up with high-performance gasoline.

## Monday

**BREAKFAST**: 8–10 egg whites and a bowl of oatmeal

**SNACK**: Bowl of assorted fruits

**SUPPLEMENTS**: Multivitamins, minerals, fish oil (T.O. am supplement pack)

**LUNCH**: 2 grilled chicken breasts with 1 baked sweet potato

**SNACK**: Bowl of fruit or salad

**SUPPLEMENTS**: Multivitamins, minerals, fish oil (T.O. pm supplement pack)

**DINNER**: 12 ounces boiled sea bass with brown rice

**SNACK**: Large salad or assorted vegetables (raw or steamed)

## Tuesday

**BREAKFAST**: 8–10 egg whites and a bowl of oatmeal

**SNACK**: Bowl of assorted fruits

**SUPPLEMENTS**: Multivitamins, minerals, fish oil (T.O. am supplement pack)

**LUNCH**: 10 ounces grilled turkey breast with 1 baked sweet potato

**SNACK**: Bowl of fruit or salad

**SUPPLEMENTS**: Multivitamins, minerals, fish oil (T.O. pm supplement pack)

**DINNER**: 12 ounces salmon with steamed white rice

**SNACK**: Large salad or assorted vegetables (raw or steamed)

## Wednesday

**BREAKFAST**: 8–10 egg whites and a bowl of oatmeal

**SNACK**: Bowl of assorted fruits

**SUPPLEMENTS**: Multivitamins, minerals, fish oil (T.O. am supplement pack)

**LUNCH**: 2 grilled chicken breasts with 1 baked sweet potato

**SNACK**: Bowl of fruit or salad

**SUPPLEMENTS**: Multivitamins, minerals, fish oil (T.O. pm supplement pack)

**DINNER**: 12 ounces sea bass with brown rice

**SNACK**: Large salad or assorted vegetables (raw or steamed)

## Thursday

**BREAKFAST**: 8–10 egg whites and a bowl of oatmeal

**SNACK**: Bowl of assorted fruits

**SUPPLEMENTS**: Multivitamins, minerals, fish oil (T.O. am supplement pack)

**LUNCH**: 10 ounces grilled turkey breast with 1 baked sweet potato

**SNACK**: Bowl of fruit or salad

**SUPPLEMENTS**: Multivitamins, minerals, fish oil (T.O. pm supplement pack)

**DINNER**: 12 ounces salmon with steamed white rice

**SNACK**: Large salad or assorted vegetables (raw or steamed)

## Friday

**BREAKFAST**: 8–10 egg whites and a bowl of oatmeal

**SNACK**: Bowl of assorted fruits

**SUPPLEMENTS**: Multivitamins, minerals, fish oil (T.O. am supplement pack)

**LUNCH**: 2 grilled chicken breasts with 1 baked sweet potato

**SNACK**: Bowl of fruit or salad

**SUPPLEMENTS**: Multivitamins, minerals, fish oil (T.O. pm supplement pack)

**DINNER**: 12 ounces sea bass with brown rice

**SNACK**: Large salad or assorted vegetables (raw or steamed)

## Saturday

**BREAKFAST**: 8–10 egg whites and a bowl of oatmeal

**SNACK**: Bowl of assorted fruits

**SUPPLEMENTS**: Multivitamins, minerals, fish oil (T.O. am supplement pack)

**LUNCH**: 10 ounces grilled turkey breast with 1 baked sweet potato

**SNACK**: Bowl of fruit or salad

**SUPPLEMENTS**: Multivitamins, minerals, fish oil (T.O. pm supplement pack)

**DINNER**: 12 ounces grilled salmon with steamed white rice

**SNACK**: Large salad or assorted vegetables (raw or steamed)

## Sunday

**BREAKFAST**: 8–10 egg whites with a bowl of oatmeal and 1 cup steamed potatoes

**SNACK**: Bowl of fruit

**SUPPLEMENTS**: Multivitamins, minerals, fish oil (T.O. pm supplement pack)

**LUNCH**: GAME

**SNACK**: GAME

**SUPPLEMENTS**: GAME

**DINNER**: 8–10 ounces grilled lean steak with 1 baked potato

**SNACK**: Steamed vegetables

I know what you're thinking after looking at this: "Does he really eat like this for four to six months?" The answer is yes!

To perform at the All-Star level, my in-season diet is rigid and disciplined. My body is like a clock—no matter what the time, the clock on the wall looks and operates the same, day in and day out. In order to make big plays, my body has to look and operate the same each day; that's why I don't change what I put into it. The only change is that as the season progresses I perform better, I'm stronger, and I reach my maximum potential.

Using my diet as a guideline, you're guaranteed to make it into the end zone. Success is yours; now go get it!

## OFF-SEASON

I exercise discipline, moderation, and common sense, even in the off-season. For the first three months after the season ends, my primary focus is recovery after such a strenuous training and dieting program. I eat fewer meals daily, and the change in schedule allows my meals to begin much later in the day and end much later at night.

## Monday

| | |
|---|---|
| 11:00–11:30 A.M. | Chicken breast and steamed potatoes |
| 2:30–3:00 P.M. | 2 small Snickers bars |
| 6:00–6:30 | Protein drink of rice milk and apple juice |
| 10:00–10:30 | Grilled salmon with salad (lettuce, tomatoes, balsamic vinegar dressing) |
| 1:00 A.M. | Small bag of Doritos chips |

## Tuesday

| | |
|---|---|
| 11:30–12:00 P.M. | Rotisserie chicken with black beans, white rice |
| 2:00 | 2–3 small bags of M&M's |
| 4:00 | Hamburger at McDonald's or Burger King |
| 6:00 | Protein drink of rice milk and apple juice |
| 8–10 | 2–3 small bags of M&M's |
| 11:00 | Sea bass and brown rice |
| 1:00 A.M. | 2 small bags of M&M's |

## Wednesday

| | |
|---|---|
| 11:00–11:30 A.M. | Chicken breast and steamed potatoes |
| 2:30–3:00 P.M. | 2 small Snickers bars |
| 6:00–6:30 | Protein drink of rice milk and apple juice |
| 10:00–10:30 | Grilled salmon with salad (lettuce, tomatoes, balsamic vinegar dressing) |
| 1:00 A.M. | Small bag of Doritos chips |

## Thursday

| | |
|---|---|
| 11:30–12:00 P.M. | Rotisserie chicken with black beans and white rice |
| 2:00 | 2 small Kit Kat bars |
| 4:00 | Hamburger at McDonald's or Burger King |
| 6:00 | Protein drink of rice milk and apple juice |
| 8:00–10:00 | 2 small Kit Kat or Snickers bars |
| 11:00 | Sea bass and brown rice |
| 1:00 A.M. | 2 small bags of M&M's |

## Friday

| | |
|---|---|
| **11:00–11:30** A.M. | Chicken breast and steamed broccoli |
| **2:30–3:00** P.M. | 2 small Snickers bars |
| **6:00–6:30** | Protein drink of rice milk and apple juice |
| **10:00–10:30** | Salmon with salad (lettuce, tomatoes, balsamic vinegar dressing) |
| **1:00** A.M. | Small bag of Ruffles chips |

## Saturday

| | |
|---|---|
| **NOON** | Rotisserie chicken with black beans and white rice |
| **4:00** P.M. | Tropical fruit smoothie made with actual tropical fruits |
| **6:00** | Mahimahi and salad |
| **9:00** | Small bag of M&M's |
| **12:00** | White wine |
| **2:00** A.M. | Salad |

## Sunday

| | |
|---|---|
| **11:00–12:00** P.M. | Pizza and salad |
| **4:00** | 1 turkey wrap with a slice of cheesecake |
| **9:00** | Salmon and salad |
| **12:00** A.M. | Small bag of potato chips |
| **12:30** | Apple martini |

I want to point out that this more laid-back diet also reflects the life of a bachelor. My days during the off-season start late and end even later. There is no such thing as nightlife from July to February, so when I do get a chance to just hang loose and kick it, I take advantage of that.

Even though I'm not big on drinking, in the midst of my travels, either on vacation or hitting the celeb scene, I may have one drink. If I do indulge, it's usually something light and clear, and definitely, as I said before, in strict moderation. True champions always drink responsibly, and they never, *ever* drink and drive. Cheers!

## THE TRUTH ABOUT SUPPLEMENTS

Because our daily diets and lifestyles often do not provide our bodies with sufficient nutrients, supplements can be an important aid to achieving optimum health. But although supplements can be a safety net, they are not a substitute for proper diet and exercise. Supplements are insurance, not replacements.

The following is for your information only and is not a recommendation; check with your doctor before beginning any supplement program.

**Vitamin A** is important for vision, bone growth, and reproduction. It helps regulate the immune system and fight off infections. Vitamin A promotes healthy surface linings of the eyes, respiratory, urinary, and intestinal tracts.

**Vitamin B1**, also known as thiamine, is vital to normal functioning of the nervous system and metabolism. It assists in the normal functions of the heart and muscles and can be found in meat, whole grains, fish, and nuts.

**Vitamin B12** acts as a coenzyme for the creation of DNA material and is important to fat, carbohydrate, and protein metabolism. It can be found in meats, fish, eggs, and dairy products.

**Vitamin C** plays a major role in numerous body functions. It is vital for a healthy immune and nervous system and as an antioxidant; it helps build collagen and enhances iron absorption.

**Vitamin D** is also known as the sunshine vitamin. Its primary function is to absorb calcium and phosphorus to aid in the development of bones and teeth, while also helping maintain a healthy nervous and immune system. It is found in many foods; some sources include fortified milk, oily fish, liver, and eggs.

**Vitamin E** protects fats, cell membranes, DNA material, and enzymes in the body against damage. It is also an antioxidant that protects against heart disease and may protect against cancer. Vitamin E can be found in many foods, including wheat germ, nuts and seeds, whole-grain cereals, eggs, and leafy greens.

**Calcium** is the most abundant mineral in the body. It is essential for normal activity of the nervous, muscular, and skeletal systems. Calcium is important for heart and kidney function and assists in blood clotting.

**Iron** is an essential component of hemoglobin, which helps transport oxygen and contributes to the storage of oxygen in the cells.

**Magnesium** contributes to bone growth and aids in the function of nerves and muscles and regulation of heart rhythm.

**Potassium** plays a role in protein synthesis and the conversion of blood sugar into glycogen. It promotes regular heartbeat and regulates the transfer of nutrients to cells.

**Omega-3 fatty acids** are found mostly in cold-water fish, such as salmon, mackerel, and halibut. They protect against coronary heart disease and may have benefit in treating arthritis.

Look for my very own supplement packs at www.tosupplements.com.

## KEY FACTS TO REMEMBER

To get the most out of your fitness program, consider the following:

- It takes a gallon of water a day to maintain fitness. Water gives you energy and helps release fat from your body. Try this: at the first sign of hunger, drink a glass of water. Oftentimes, the body confuses hunger and thirst and can be satisfied with a glass of $H_2O$.

- Crash Diets are dangerous! You cannot lose weight by starving. Five, six, or even seven small, healthy meals a day will keep your metabolism going. Eating sensibly, not starving, will help burn fat and keep the pounds off.

- The time you take to rest is as important as the time you take to train. Work smart, not just hard.

The more information you have, the more successful you will be in planning your fitness program. Use the information in these chapters as guidelines to prepare the plan that best fits your lifestyle, your objectives, and your schedule. With discipline, moderation, and commitment, you will be able to achieve your fitness goals!

# PART IV

# Intro to Fitness:
# The Body and the Bands

've always looked for ways to improve or perfect my workout, primarily because I believe the body is designed to do remarkable things. I'm always ready to push myself to the next level of training to ensure that with each day, I'm getting stronger and better.

Although I was introduced to resistance bands early on in my career, I never thought to use them the way I use them now.

After I sustained the injury to my leg in 2005, my friend and team trainer Alex McKechnie had to develop a way for me to work out with resistance without using free weights or weight machines. That mission seemed impossible.

Then the simple answer came to us: instead of weights, I'd use my body. I was 224 pounds of solid muscle. Was this heavy enough to achieve what I needed to? Absolutely! We just had to figure out how I could become my own weight.

Band training was the best option. In fact, strength-band training has been around for more than one hundred years. Bands allow you to train your body from any angle with perfect and smooth tension, using your body's own weight. Using the bands, my entire body had to work to perform a single exercise. When I was working to strengthen my legs, for example, I had to use all parts of my body; every muscle got stronger. The results were amazing, and I got a new perspective on working out.

Bands, especially my version, give new definition to strength training. You are your resistance. Before using bands, I never knew my own strength. It's funny, because I now understand what that means. Not only can I lift 224 pounds with ease, I can now perform at levels I was never able to before.

The following sections are dedicated to the individuals who throughout my career have helped me achieve maximum results at times when things seemed hopeless. I've taken the knowledge given to me by Rick Renner, Britt Brown, Eric Sugarman, John Paterson, Alex McKechnie, Jim Cotta, Hank Sloan, Tim Gurley, Chelsea England,

Carol McMakin, Brian Bureynski, Tim McKelroy, and Jasén Powell and designed the next level of muscle and sports-specific exercises guaranteed to give you an All-Star body.

Although I still believe in traditional forms of weight training, bands have become one of my favorite forms of working out.

I truly believe that the strength channeled during each exercise with the bands helps to improve our quality of life overall.

This is more than just exercise; it's about building a body that will ultimately help build a better and stronger you.

For more on my bands visit www.tobands.com.

---

# 8

# How I Find Fitness

**Songs are an instrumental** part of my workout and everyday routine. With certain songs, the message is so precise that I find myself listening to the song over and over again. I feel the same way about a really good book; there are just certain things you need to read more than once.

When it came time for me to choose a song for my website, I hit many roadblocks. Rather than jump through all the legal hoops to use someone else's song, I headed to my studio and recorded my own song. "I'm Back" was released when I signed with Dallas. This was my third and, I hoped final team, and I needed something that would really speak to who I was and what it takes to be me—an All-Star athlete playing at an elite level.

Finding fitness for me means never giving up. It means showing up inspired in spite of adversity and challenges. It means performing like a champion and giving 100 percent each and every day.

I've performed hurt, I've performed broken, I've performed bruised—mentally, physically, and emotionally. Through it all, I've performed at top level.

I've found a new level of fitness every day, challenging myself to get stronger and better, never accepting defeat, even in the midst of defeat.

Fitness is more than physical, it is melding of the mind, body, and soul. I work my mind by taking in positive information and learning as much as I can every day. I dedicate forty-five minutes each day to reading and learning something new.

I work my body, dedicating at least forty-five minutes to physical exercise and challenging myself once a week by increasing the intensity in some area of my workout to become better and stronger.

I work my spirit by allowing my faith to lead me to my destiny, never allowing my fears to overshadow my actions. I've learned to stay in the game, even if I do become afraid, because my faith is the key to accomplishing my goals.

I find fitness by trusting myself, believing in myself, and proving to myself that I matter. Life is truly worth living if you realize that no matter where you came from or where you are now, you have the ability to change.

Finding fitness is believing in change and knowing that no matter the odds against you, you can find fitness for yourself.

---

### T.O. TESTIMONY: *The Making of a Champion*

I've had so many moments that have defined my life and made me feel like a winner. Yet there have been rare moments when I've actually felt like a champion.

On April 1, 2003, I had an opportunity to speak to the U.S. Senate regarding a cause that is near and dear to my heart. I was able to speak on behalf of my grandmother, Alice Black, who is suffering from Alzheimer's. My grandmother has always been my champion. Below is an excerpt from my speech. Each word and thought represents how I was able to testify on behalf of her and millions of others and help make a difference for a worthy cause:

#### From the 15th Annual Alzheimer's Association Public Policy Forum, Washington, D.C., April 1, 2003

Good morning, Senator Specter and Senator Harkin. I am honored to be here. My name is Terrell Owens. I am here to talk to you about an incredible woman named Alice Black. Alice is my grandmother, and she has Alzheimer's disease. While I'm here in Washington, she is in a nursing home in Talladega, Alabama. At this point, she remembers mainly me, her late husband, and the woman who is here with me today, Marilyn Heard, her daughter and my mother.

Professionally, I have achieved one of my dreams: I play football in the National Football League. I am a wide receiver for the San Francisco 49ers.

In my seven seasons in the NFL, I have caught hundreds of passes, scored many touchdowns, set numerous 49er and NFL records, and have been to the Pro Bowl three times. Despite this success, I am basically powerless to help a woman that I love very dearly. . . . Football has provided me with a certain amount of fame and privilege; however, no amount of fame or privilege can heal my grandmother. While I gladly pay her medical and health care expenses, I cannot change the fact that she has Alzheimer's and continues to suffer.

One of the real tragedies of Alzheimer's is the isolation it produces. The woman who helped raise me is barely aware of my accomplishments or my position in life. I am proud to be Alice Black's grandson, and I simply wish that she was able to celebrate what we have become, where we are going, all the while remembering where we have been. During 2002, I had the honor of serving as the celebrity team chair for the Alzheimer's Association Northern California & Northern Nevada Memory Walk. I plan to serve again this year as the celebrity chair for the 2003 Memory Walk. . . .

I know there are millions of others who have suffered with a loved one stricken with Alzheimer's, just as my family and I have suffered. I am truly humbled to have been chosen to represent many of those persons here today. I believe I speak for all of us when I ask this committee to help us help those who cannot help themselves.

Unfortunately, I cannot go out and make a big play or score a touchdown that will cure my grandmother and the millions of others who suffer from Alzheimer's. However, I am here today as part of a team that can work together to defeat Alzheimer's. I am asking the senators on this committee and President Bush to help me, Coach Martz, and the millions of persons we represent to team with us to defeat Alzheimer's. Together, we can make a difference and defeat this horrible disease once and for all.

# PART V

# Champion!

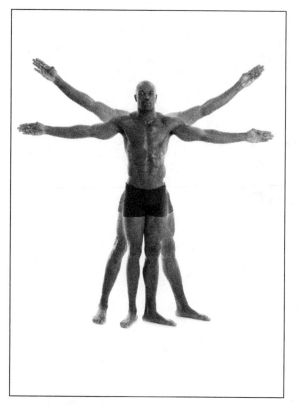

This section of the book is for the true champion and physical warrior. In each of the following chapters, I'm going to show you how to blow out your arms, legs, chest, shoulders, back, and abs as never before. Getting through this means you're ready to become an MVP for life. We're about to build your stats with this section, baby!

These workouts will train your muscles to all-new levels in just 8⅛ minutes each. Each 8⅛-minute workout contains three exercises that you perform one after another in a circuit. To complete the champion workout, you will need to finish three circuits in a row. For the maximum workout, I've designed each one of these workouts using my bands; however, you can use any form of resistance.

## General Information

**Frequency:** 2 times per week; for example, Tuesday and Friday

**Warm-up and cool-down:** 5 minutes of light cardiovascular work: riding an exercise bike, walking on a treadmill, light jogging, or walking in place

**Sets:** 1 set per exercise per circuit

**Repetitions (reps) per set:** 30

**Rep speed:** Your rep speed for this program is different from that of all other programs. In order to create champion-caliber muscle groups, you will want to implement a 1 count (say "one-Mississippi" in your head) during the positive stage of the movement and a 3 count (say "one-Mississippi, two-Mississippi, three-Mississippi" in your head) during the negative stage.

**Breathing:** Be sure to exhale during the positive stage of the movement.

## CHAMPION WORKOUT INSTRUCTIONS

These workouts will train your muscles to all-new levels in just $8\frac{1}{8}$ minutes. Each $8\frac{1}{8}$-minute workout contains 3 exercises that you perform in sequence to complete a circuit. The goal is to get through 3 sets of each circuit.

### General information:

Perform the exercises in order.

Here's how your champion workout should look:

| Perform circuit | Repeat circuit: | Repeat circuit: |
| --- | --- | --- |
| exercise 1 | exercise 1 | exercise 1 |
| exercise 2 | exercise 2 | exercise 2 |
| exercise 3 | exercise 3 | exercise 3 |

### Cool-down

5 minutes of light cardiovascular exercise: riding an exercise bike, walking on a treadmill, doing jumping jacks, jogging, or walking in place; just remember that it is a "cooldown," so you want to keep the exertion level low.

**9**

# Champion Arms

*You don't get arms like these by just eating spinach! Popeye don't have nothing on me.*

— TERRELL OWENS

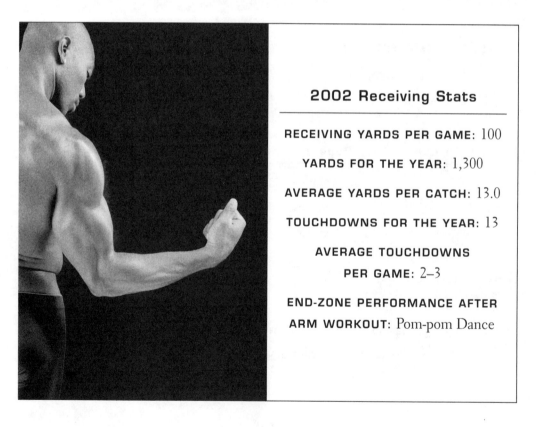

## 2002 Receiving Stats

**RECEIVING YARDS PER GAME:** 100

**YARDS FOR THE YEAR:** 1,300

**AVERAGE YARDS PER CATCH:** 13.0

**TOUCHDOWNS FOR THE YEAR:** 13

**AVERAGE TOUCHDOWNS PER GAME:** 2–3

**END-ZONE PERFORMANCE AFTER ARM WORKOUT:** Pom-pom Dance

# Exercise 1. Standing Arms-up Biceps Curls

**Muscle group targeted:** Biceps (front of arms)

**SETUP/STARTING POSITION:** Anchor a band at chest height and position your body facing the anchor point. Grip a handle in each hand and raise your arms until they are parallel with the floor. Rotate your wrists so that your palms are facing up. Move away from the anchor point. You should be far enough from the anchor point that there is a slight amount of tension on the band. Keep your feet and knees hip-width apart.

**MOVEMENT:**

**Positive Stage:** Pull the handles toward your face until your forearms are just past perpendicular to the floor.

**Negative Stage:** At a controlled speed, lower your hands to the starting position.

> **Buddy's Tip** Tighten your stomach muscles and push your buttocks forward and upward. Try to keep your elbows stationary; do not move them up or down as you pull.

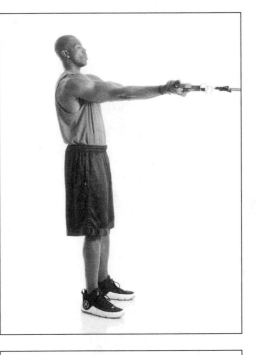

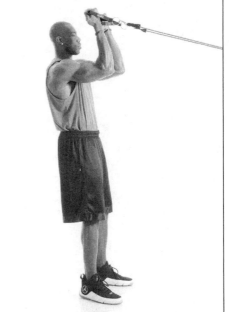

## Exercise 2. Triceps Press-downs

**Muscle group targeted:** Triceps (back of arms)

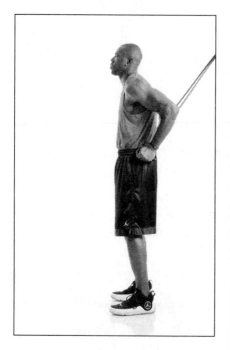

**SETUP/STARTING POSITION:** Anchor a band above your head. Position your body so that your back is to the anchor point. Grip a handle in each hand and push them down so that your palms are resting on your hips. Your elbows should be behind your body and shoulder-width apart.

**MOVEMENT:**

**Positive Stage:** Push the handles straight down until your arms are almost fully extended.

**Negative Stage:** At a controlled speed, return your hands to the starting position.

**Buddy's Tip** Stabilize your body by tightening your stomach muscles and pushing your buttocks forward and upward. Be sure to keep your shoulders down throughout the movement.

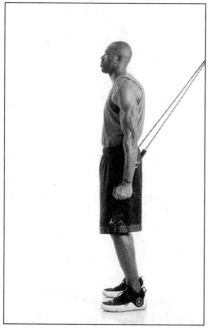

# Exercise 3. Standing Rotating Curls

**Muscle group targeted:** Biceps (front of arms)

**SETUP/STARTING POSITION:** Stand on a band with your feet hip-width apart. Make sure that the length of the band from the outside of your shoes to the handles is the same on both sides. Grip a handle in each hand and stand up straight. Your arms should be straight down at your sides with your palms turned in, resting on your thighs. Keep your knees slightly bent.

**MOVEMENT:**

**Positive Stage:** Rotate and raise the handles until they are at chest height with your palms facing up.

**Negative Stage:** At a controlled speed, lower the handles to the starting position.

> **Buddy's Tip** Try to keep your elbows in one place; avoid moving your elbows forward or backward excessively as you raise the handles.

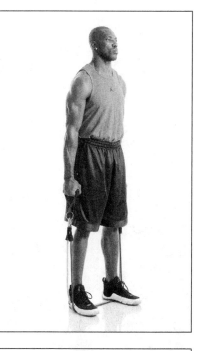

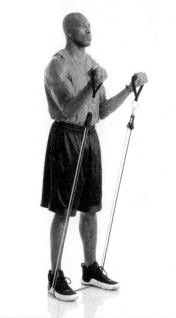

# 10

# Champion Chest

*If Superman can wear an "S" on his chest, maybe I'll get a "T" for me.*

— TERRELL OWENS

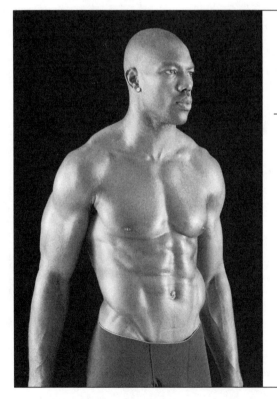

### 1998 Receiving Stats

**RECEIVING YARDS PER GAME:** 67

**YARDS FOR THE YEAR:** 1,097

**AVERAGE YARDS PER CATCH:** 16.4

**TOUCHDOWNS FOR THE YEAR:** 14

**END-ZONE PERFORMANCE AFTER CHEST WORKOUT:** Souljah Boy Dance

# Exercise 1. Two-Arm Low Chest Press

**Muscle group targeted:** Pectoralis major (chest)

**SETUP/STARTING POSITION:** Anchor a band at waist height. Turn your back to the anchor point and grip a handle in each hand. The band should be under your arm. Move away from the anchor point so that there is a slight amount of tension on the band. Place one foot ahead of the other and lean forward a little. Keep your elbows up and your hands shoulder-width apart with your palms facing down.

**MOVEMENT:**

**Positive Stage:** Push the handles forward and together until they are at eye level and your arms are almost fully extended.

**Negative Stage:** At a controlled speed, return the handles to the starting position.

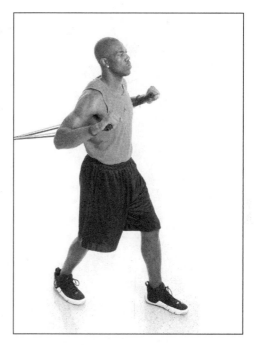

> **Buddy's Tip**  Right before you push the handles out for the first rep, tighten your stomach muscles and push your buttocks forward and upward.

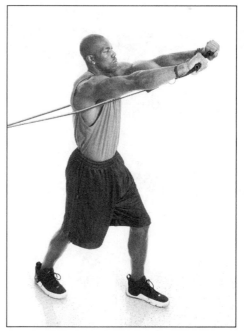

## Excercise 2. Two-Arm Forward Chest Press

**Muscle group targeted:** Pectoralis major (chest)

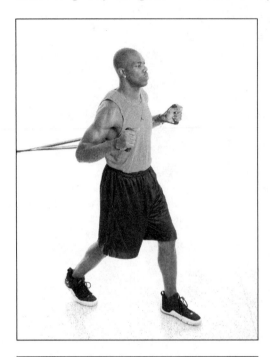

**SETUP/STARTING POSITION:** Anchor a band at chest height. Turn your back to the anchor point and grip a handle in each hand. Move away from the anchor point so that there is a slight amount of tension on the band. Place one foot ahead of the other and lean forward a little. Keep your elbows up and your hands shoulder-width apart with your hands facing in.

**MOVEMENT:**

**Positive Stage:** Push the handles forward and slightly in until they are at eye level and your arms are almost fully extended.

**Negative Stage:** At a controlled speed, return the handles to the starting position.

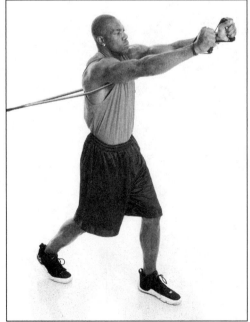

**Buddy's Tips** This exercise needs a strong and balanced center. Right before you push the handles out for the first rep, tighten your stomach muscles and push your buttocks forward and upward.

# Exercise 3. Kneeling One-Arm Chest Fly

**Muscle group targeted:** Pectoralis major (chest)

**SETUP/STARTING POSITION:** Anchor a band at waist height. Grip both handles with your right hand and turn your body so that your right shoulder is facing the anchor point. Position your right arm out to the side so that it is parallel with the floor. Rotate your wrist so that your thumb is on top. Kneel on the floor. Your distance from the anchor point should be enough that there is a slight amount of tension on the band. Keep your left hand on your left hip and your chest up.

**MOVEMENT:**

**Positive Stage:** Pull the handle out and across your body until it is just past the center of your chest.

**Negative Stage:** At a controlled speed, return the handle to the starting position.

Complete the desired number of reps and then switch sides.

> **Buddy's Tip** Tighten your stomach muscles and pull your buttocks upward and forward. Do not bend your working arm too much as you pull the handle across your body. If you find that your arm is bending excessively, try decreasing the amount of resistance.

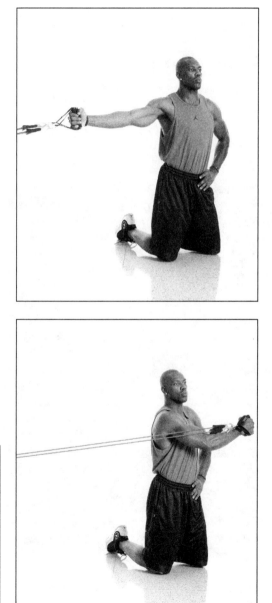

# 11

# Champion Legs

*I don't play to make history, yet I make plays that do.*

— Terrell Owens

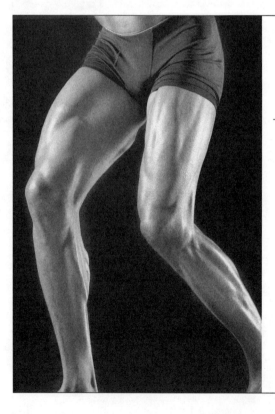

## 2004 Receiving Stats

**RECEIVING YARDS PER GAME:** 77

**YARDS FOR THE YEAR:** 1,200

**AVERAGE YARDS PER CATCH:** 15.6

**TOUCHDOWNS FOR THE YEAR:** 14

**END-ZONE PERFORMANCE
AFTER LEG WORKOUT:**
Sharpie Time, Baby!

# Exercise 1. Squats

**Muscle group targeted:** Quadriceps and gluteals (thighs and buttocks)

**SETUP/STARTING POSITION:** Anchor a band at floor height. Face the anchor point and grip a handle in each hand. Stand up straight and raise the handles to shoulder height. Rotate your palms so that they are facing forward. Your knees and feet should be hip-width apart.

**MOVEMENT:**

**Negative Stage:** At a controlled speed, squat down until your thighs are parallel with the floor.

**Positive Stage:** Push from your heels and raise your body until your legs are almost straight.

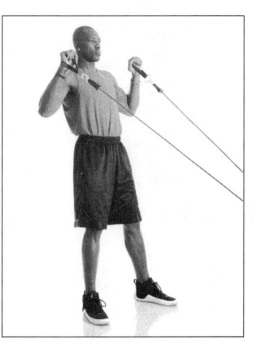

> **Buddy's Tip**  This exercise will add a new element to the squat because the bands are out in front of you. Start the negative stage of the movement by sticking out your buttocks, similar to the motion required for sitting in a chair. Make sure that your knees are not pushing in toward each other or bowing out. If this is the case, decrease the resistance. Keep your chest up during the whole movement.

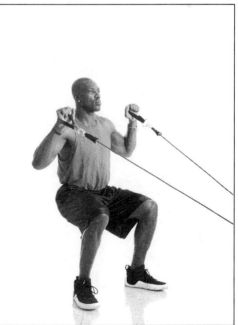

## Exercise 2. Lunge

**Muscle group targeted:** Quadriceps and gluteals (thighs and buttocks)

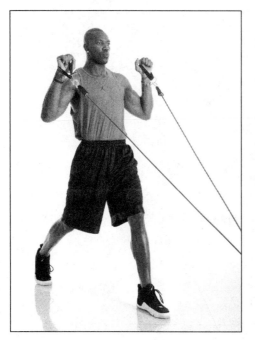

**SETUP/STARTING POSITION:** Anchor a band at floor level. Face the anchor point and position your legs with your left foot forward. Grip a handle in each hand and raise the handles to shoulder height. Rotate your palms so that they are facing forward.

**MOVEMENT:**

**Negative Stage:** At a controlled speed, lower your body straight down until your left thigh is parallel with the floor.

**Positive Stage:** Push from your left heel and raise your body until your left leg is almost straight.

Complete the desired number of reps and then switch sides.

**Buddy's Tip** The knee of your front leg should not move forward during the exercise. To avoid this, concentrate on lowering your hips straight down to the floor.

# Exercise 3. Resisted Leg Curl

**Muscle group targeted:** Hamstrings (back of legs)

**SETUP/STARTING POSITION:** Anchor a band at floor height. Face the anchor point and wrap an ankle strap around the middle of each foot. Place your hands on your hips and keep your head straight.

**MOVEMENT:**

**Positive Stage:** Push your left heel back and up until your shin is parallel with the floor.

**Negative Stage:** At a controlled pace, lower your heel to the starting position. Complete the desired number of reps and then switch sides.

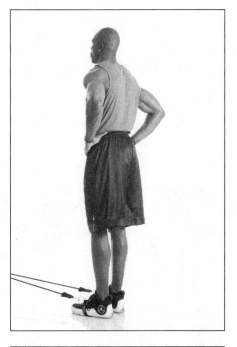

> **Buddy's Tip** Right before you perform your first rep, tighten your stomach muscles and push your buttocks forward and upward. It is important that you do not move your thigh too far forward as you push your heel back.

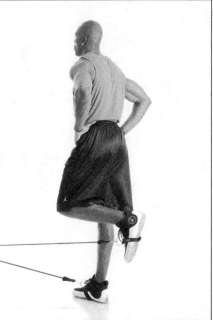

# 12

# Champion Shoulders

*Impossible is not an option.*

—Terrell Owens

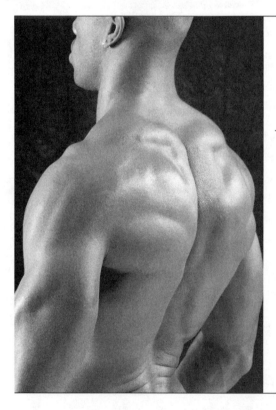

## 2000 Receiving Stats

RECEIVING YARDS PER GAME: 97

YARDS FOR THE YEAR: 1,451

AVERAGE YARDS PER CATCH: 15.0

TOUCHDOWNS FOR THE YEAR: 13

END-ZONE PERFORMANCE
AFTER SHOULDER WORKOUT: T.O.

# Exercise 1. Front Shoulder Raise

**Muscle group targeted:** Anterior deltoid (front of shoulders)

**SETUP/STARTING POSITION:** Step on a band with your feet hip-width apart. Make sure that the length of the band from the outside of your shoe to the handle is the same on both sides. Grip a handle in each hand and stand up straight with your knees slightly bent. Your arms should be almost fully extended with your hands in front of your thighs. Rotate your wrists so that your palms are facing toward your legs.

**MOVEMENT:**

**Positive Stage:** Raise your arms until they are parallel with the floor.

**Negative Stage:** At a controlled speed, lower your arms to the starting position.

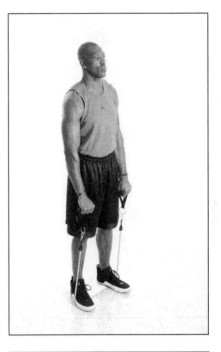

> **Buddy's Tip** Tighten your stomach and pull your buttocks forward and upward. When you raise the handles, try not to bend your arms too deeply and keep your hands shoulder-width apart.

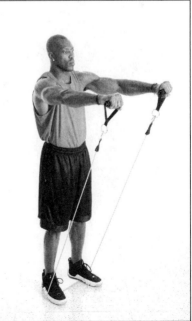

## Exercise 2. Standing Lateral Raise

**Muscle group targeted:** Medial deltoid (middle shoulder)

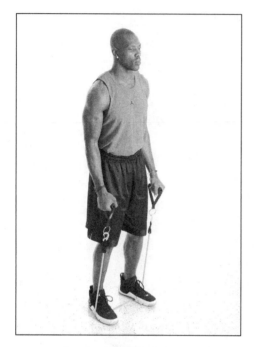

**SETUP/STARTING POSITION:** Stand on a band with your feet hip-width apart. Make sure that the length of the band from the outside of your shoe to the handle is the same on both sides. Reach down and grip a handle in each hand. Stand up straight with your arms at your sides and your palms facing toward each other. Keep your knees slightly bent.

**MOVEMENT:**

**Positive Stage:** Raise your arms straight out to the sides until your elbows reach shoulder height.

**Negative Stage:** At a controlled speed, lower your arms to the starting position.

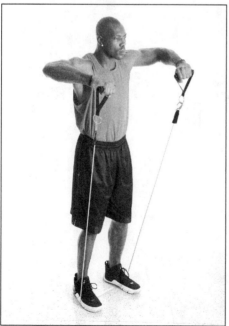

**Buddy's Tip** Tighten your stomach muscles and pull your buttocks forward and upward. Keep your elbows higher than your hands as you raise your arms. A great trick to help you use proper form is to imagine that you are pouring milk out of cartons as you raise your arms.

# Exercise 3. Front Shoulder Press

**Muscle group targeted:** Anterior deltoid (front shoulder)

**SETUP/STARTING POSITION:** Stand on the middle of a band with your right foot and grip a handle in each hand. Stand up straight and place your left foot behind you. Raise the handles to shoulder height and rotate your wrists so that your palms are facing forward. Keep a slight bend in your right leg. Your hands should be shoulder-width apart.

**MOVEMENT:**

**Positive Stage:** Push the handles straight up and over your head until your arms are almost fully extended.

**Negative Stage:** At a controlled speed, lower your hands to the starting position.

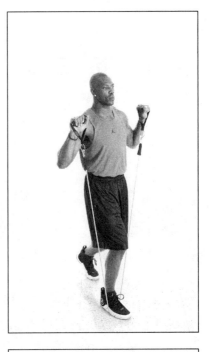

> **Buddy's Tip** Stabilize your lower body by tightening your stomach muscles and pushing your buttocks forward and upward.

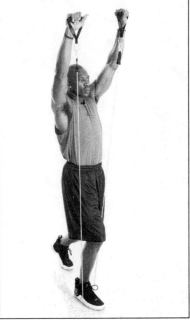

# 13

# Champion Back

*Is there anyone better than me? Nope!*

— TERRELL OWENS

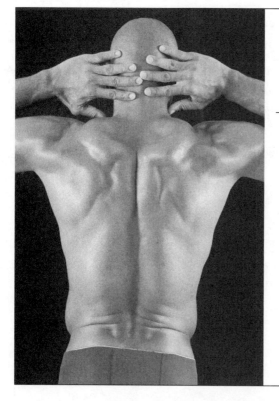

## 2006 Receiving Stats

**RECEIVING YARDS PER GAME:** 85

**YARDS FOR THE YEAR:** 1,180

**AVERAGE YARDS PER CATCH:** 13.9

**TOUCHDOWNS FOR THE YEAR:** 13

**END-ZONE PERFORMANCE
AFTER BACK WORKOUT:** Camera
time — I'm ready for my close-up!

# Exercise 1. Standing Lat Pull

**Muscle group targeted:** Latissimus dorsi (middle and outer back)

**SETUP/STARTING POSITION:** Anchor a band at chest height. Position your body so that you are facing the anchor point and grip a handle in each hand. Your arms should be out in front of you, parallel with the floor and almost fully extended. Rotate your hands so that your palms are facing down. Move far enough away from the anchor point that there is a slight amount of tension on the band. Bend forward at the waist, keeping your chest up.

**MOVEMENT:**

**Positive Stage:** Keeping your elbows up, pull the handles straight back until your hands are right in front of your shoulders.

**Negative Stage:** At a controlled speed, return your hands to the starting position.

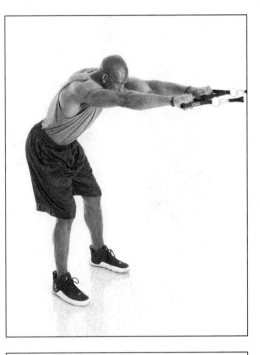

> **Buddy's Tip** Tighten your stomach muscles and push your buttocks forward and upward. To isolate the back muscles, hold the handles with a closed but loose grip.

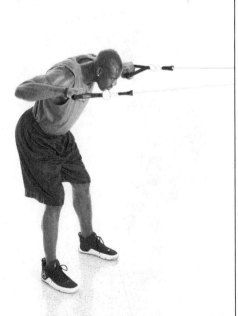

## Exercise 2. Standing Back Rows

**Muscle group targeted:** Latissimus dorsi (middle and outer back)

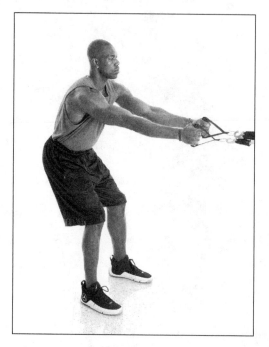

**SETUP/STARTING POSITION:** Anchor a band at waist height. Position your body so that you are facing the anchor point and grip a handle in each hand. Your arms should be straight out in front of you, parallel with the floor. Rotate your hands so that your thumbs are on top. Move far enough away from the anchor point that there is a slight amount of tension on the band. Keep your knees and feet hip-width apart.

**MOVEMENT:**

**Positive Stage:** Keeping your elbows down and your arms tight to your body, pull the handles back to your stomach.

**Negative Stage:** At a controlled speed, return the handles to the starting position.

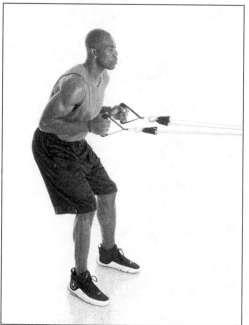

> **Buddy's Tip** Create the pelvic tilt by tightening your stomach muscles and pushing your buttocks forward and upward. To isolate the back muscles, hold the handles with a closed but loose grip.

# Exercise 3. Forward Lat Extension

**Muscle group targeted:** Latissimus dorsi (middle and outer back)

**SETUP/STARTING POSITION:** Anchor a band at chest height. Position your body so that you are facing the anchor point and grip a handle in each hand. Your arms should be out in front of you, parallel with the floor and almost fully extended. Rotate your hands so that your palms are facing in toward each other. Move far enough away from the anchor point that there is a slight amount of tension on the band. Keep your knees and feet hip-width apart.

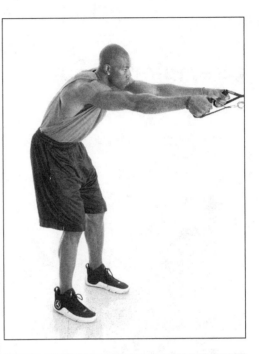

**MOVEMENT:**

**Positive Stage:** Pull the handles forward and down until your hands are just past your thighs.

**Negative Stage:** At a controlled speed, return your hands to the starting position.

> **Buddy's Tip** Incorporate the pelvic tilt into your stance: tighten your stomach muscles and move your buttocks forward and upward. As you pull the handles, do not bend your arms too much; they should be bent only slightly throughout the exercise.

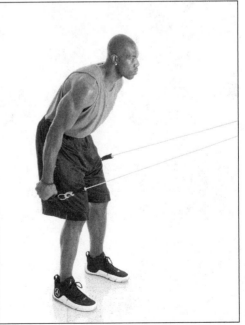

# 14

# Champion Core

*They tell me to be more politically correct. I'm not a politician, I'm a ballplayer.*

—Terrell Owens

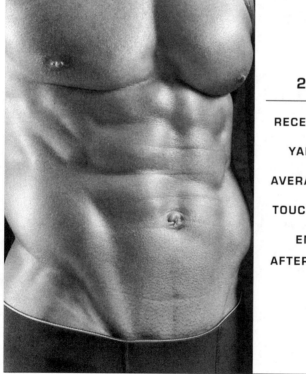

## 2007 Receiving Stats

**RECEIVING YARDS PER GAME:** 81

**YARDS FOR THE YEAR:** 1,355

**AVERAGE YARDS PER CATCH:** 16.7

**TOUCHDOWNS FOR THE YEAR:** 15

**END-ZONE PERFORMANCE AFTER CORE WORKOUT:** Popcorn to the crowd!

# Exercise 1. Kneeling Ab Crunch

**SETUP/STARTING POSITION:** In a standing position, anchor a band above your head. Position your body so that you are facing the anchor point and grip a handle in each hand. Kneel down with your knees close together and hold the handles right in front of your head. Rotate your hands so that your palms are facing in toward each other. Keep your elbows in.

**MOVEMENT:**

**Positive Stage:** Crunch down and lower your upper body until your elbows touch your thighs.

**Negative Stage:** At a controlled pace, raise your upper body and handles to the starting position.

> **Buddy's Tip**   Your arms should be relaxed; hold the handles with a closed but loose grip.

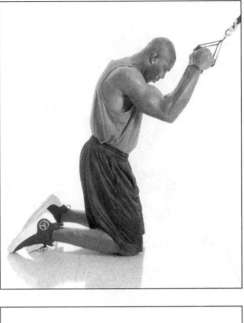

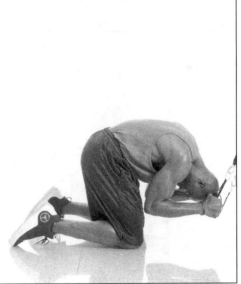

## Exercise 2. Kneeling Alternating Ab Crunch

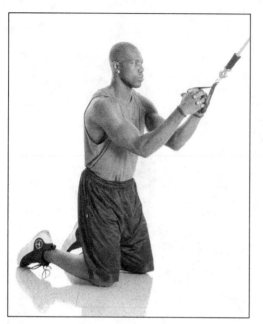

**SETUP/STARTING POSITION:** In a standing position, anchor a band above your head. Position your body so that you are facing the anchor point and grip both handles together with both hands. Kneel down with your knees close together and hold the handles right in front of your head. Keep your elbows in.

**MOVEMENT:**

**Positive Stage:** Crunch down until your elbows touch your left knee.

**Negative Stage:** At a controlled pace, raise your upper body and the handles to the starting position.

**Positive Stage:** Crunch down until your elbows touch your right knee.

**Negative Stage:** At a controlled pace, raise your upper body and the handles to the starting position.

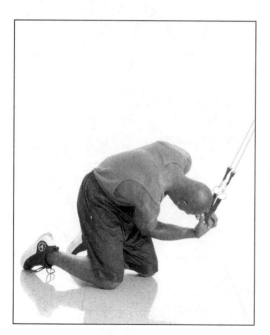

> **Buddy's Tip** Your arms should be relaxed; hold the handles with a closed but loose grip.

# Exercise 3. High-Low Wood Chop

**SETUP/STARTING POSITION:** In a standing position, anchor a band above your head. Grip the handle (or handles) with both hands and turn your body so that your left shoulder faces the anchor point. Raise the handle up and to the left side so that it is at ear height. Your arms should be up and almost fully extended. Move far enough away from the anchor point that there is a slight amount of tension on the band. Keep your feet shoulder-width apart.

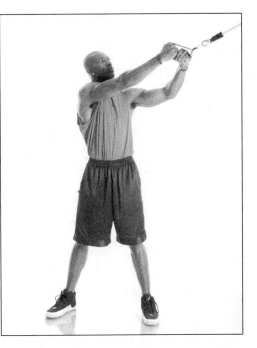

**MOVEMENT:**

**Positive Stage:** Pull the handle down and across your body until it is just past your right knee.

**Negative Stage:** At a controlled speed, return the handle to the starting position. Complete the desired number of reps and then switch sides.

> **Buddy's Tip** Remember that this is not an arm exercise. Concentrate on using your stomach muscles to pull the handle down and across your body. Your arms should be bent only slightly throughout the exercise.

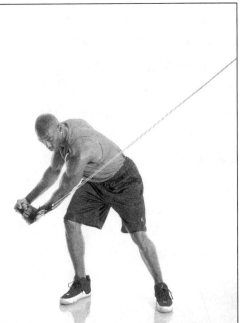

---

# 15

# Sports-Specific Workouts

**For years I've wanted** to design workouts that were so sports-specific they would help athletes of any kind advance their game to the next level.

As a lover of many sports, I've not only devised muscle-strengthening exercises that will enhance any athlete's game, I've also created exercises that will teach young athletes how to strengthen not only the major muscle groups but the supporting muscle groups so that they can perform on an elite level.

Each sport has a different exercise workout routine because the moves required for each sport vary. Although I haven't mastered each sport as well as I've mastered football, I believe that we can learn to dominate any and every game we set our minds to.

Follow the guidelines at the beginning of each sport workout, and be consistent. As the weeks progress, you will be amazed at how much better you perform. Before you begin your first workout, tell your opponents to "Watch out and getcha popcorn ready!" because your game is about to be raised to an all-new level.

## General Information

For these programs you should keep the number of reps high, so that you increase your speed and strength without losing flexibility.

Perform the exercises in order. Complete the desired number of sets per exercise and then move on to the next exercise.

# BASEBALL

**FAVORITE BASEBALL PLAYER**: *A-Rod is cool; however, Barry Bonds is, and always has been, the man.*

Baseball is a sport that requires swinging, throwing, running, and shuffling. The exercises in this routine are designed to strengthen all the muscles required for those movements. Follow the guidelines below and watch your game performance take off!

## Program Guidelines

**Frequency:** 3 times per week: for example, Monday, Wednesday, and Friday.

**Warm-up and cool-down:** 5 minutes of light cardiovascular work: riding an exercise bike, walking on a treadmill, light jogging, or walking in place

**Sets:** 3 per exercise

**Repetitions (reps) per set:** 15

**Rep speed:** Use a 1 count (say "one-Mississippi" in your head) during the positive stage of the movement and a 2 count (say "one-Mississippi, two-Mississippi" in your head) during the negative stage.

**Breathing:** Be sure to exhale during the positive stage of the movement.

## Making Progress

Keep in mind that you will need to adjust the resistance so that you are struggling on the last rep of your targeted rep number. This will ensure that you get the full benefit from every set.

## Exercise 1. Infield Quick Side Throw

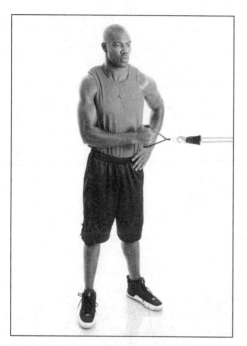

**SETUP/STARTING POSITION:** Anchor a band at stomach height. Position your body so that your left shoulder is facing the anchor point. Grip the handle with your right hand and place it against your stomach right below your ribs. Your right forearm should be parallel with the floor. Move your body far enough from the anchor point that there is a slight amount of tension on the band. Keep your feet shoulder-width apart and place your left hand on your left hip.

**MOVEMENT:**

**Positive Stage:** Keep your upper right arm tight against your body and rotate your forearm out and to the side, until your arm stops naturally.

**Negative Stage:** At a controlled speed, rotate your forearm back to the starting position.

Complete the desired number of reps and then switch sides.

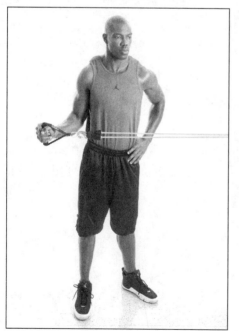

**Buddy's Tip** The pelvic tilt will automatically place many of your joints in the correct position. Tighten your stomach muscles and push your buttocks forward and upward. As you perform the exercise, imagine that you are giving a quick toss to your teammate to tag an opponent out.

# Exercise 2. Overhead Catch

**SETUP/STARTING POSITION:** Anchor a band at chest height. Position your body so that you are facing the anchor point. Grip the handle with your right hand and raise it out to the side so that your arm is parallel with the floor. Your elbow should be bent, creating a 90-degree angle between your forearm and upper arm. Move your body far enough from the anchor point that there is a slight amount of tension on the band. Position your feet shoulder-width apart and rest your left hand on your left hip.

**MOVEMENT:**

**Positive Stage:** Pull the handle and rotate your arm up, until your arm stops naturally.

**Negative Stage:** At a controlled speed, rotate your arm back to the starting position.

Complete the desired number of reps and than switch sides.

> **Buddy's Tip** Create the pelvic tilt by tightening your stomach muscles and pushing your buttocks forward and upward. As you rotate your arm and pull the handle up, try not to move your upper arm forward or backward; keep it straight out to the side.

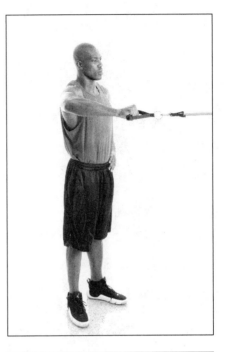

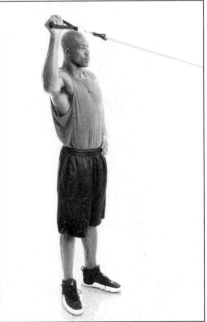

## Exercise 3. Power Swing

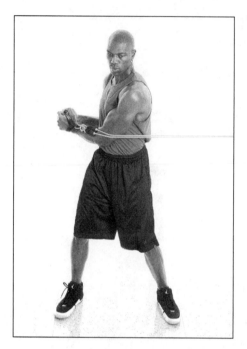

**SETUP/STARTING POSITION:** Anchor a band at stomach height. Grip the handle (or handles) with both hands and turn your body so that your left shoulder faces the anchor point. Move far enough away from the anchor point that there is a slight amount of tension on the band. Hold the handle tight to your stomach, just below your ribs. Keep your feet shoulder-width apart and your knees slightly bent.

**MOVEMENT:**

**Positive Stage:** Twist your upper body to the right until it stops naturally.

**Negative Stage:** At a controlled speed, return your upper body to the starting position.

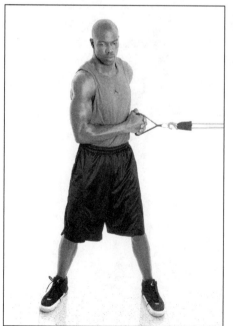

**Buddy's Tip** One of the most important muscle groups for a powerful swing is the core (stomach) muscles; this exercise is designed to strengthen your core muscles. Tighten your stomach muscles and push your buttocks forward and upward. Concentrate on using only your stomach muscles to twist your body; your arms should not do any of the work.

## Exercise 4. Infield Ground Ball Shuffle

**SETUP/STARTING POSITION:** Anchor a band at waist height. Position your body so that you are facing the anchor and grip a handle in each hand. Keep your arms out in front of your body with the handles at chest height. Move far enough away from the anchor point that there is a slight amount of tension on the band. Your knees should be shoulder-width apart and slightly bent.

**MOVEMENT:** Shuffle your feet to the right side with small lateral steps until you have traveled 3 to 4 feet. Then shuffle your feet to the left side with small lateral steps back to the starting position.

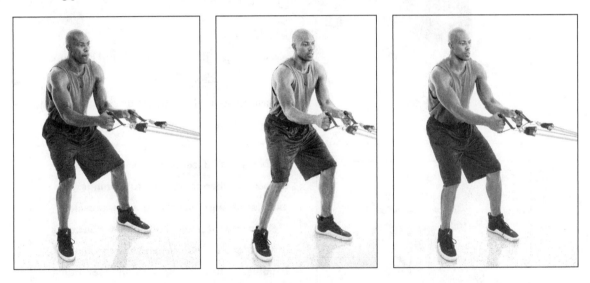

**Buddy's Tip**  Right before you shuffle, tighten your stomach muscles and push your buttocks forward and upward.

## Exercise 5. Front Ball Catch

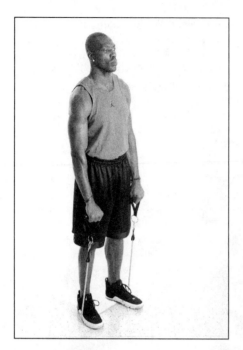

**SETUP/STARTING POSITION:** Stand on a band with your feet hip-width apart. Make sure that the length of the band from the outside of your shoe to the handle is the same on both sides. Grip a handle in each hand and stand up straight with your knees slightly bent. Your arms should be almost fully extended, with your hands in front of your thighs. Rotate your wrists so that your palms are facing toward your legs.

**MOVEMENT:**

**Positive Stage:** Raise your arms until they are parallel with the floor.

**Negative Stage:** At a controlled speed, lower your arms to the starting position.

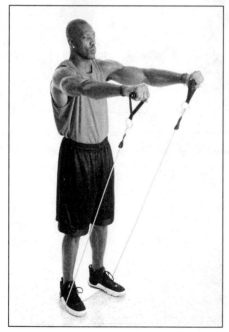

**Buddy's Tip** Baseball games can be long, especially when there are extra innings. This exercise strengthens the shoulder muscles. Tighten your stomach and pull your buttocks forward and upward. When you raise the handles, try not to bend your arms too much, and keep your hands shoulder-width apart.

# Exercise 6. Power Throw

**SETUP/STARTING POSITION:** Anchor a band above your head. Grip the handle (or handles) with both hands and turn your body so that your left shoulder faces the anchor point. Raise the handle up and to the left side so that it is at ear height. Your arms should be up and almost fully extended. Move far enough away from the anchor point that there is a slight amount of tension on the band. Keep your feet shoulder-width apart.

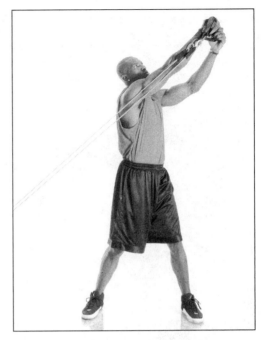

**MOVEMENT:**

**Positive Stage:** Pull the handle down and across your body until it is just past your right knee.

**Negative Stage:** At a controlled speed, return the handle to the starting position.

Complete the desired number of reps and then switch sides.

> **Buddy's Tip** This exercise is designed to build strength in the stomach muscles that are used to pitch and throw. Remember that this is not an arm exercise; concentrate on using your stomach muscles to pull the handle down and across your body. Your arms should be only slightly bent throughout the exercise.

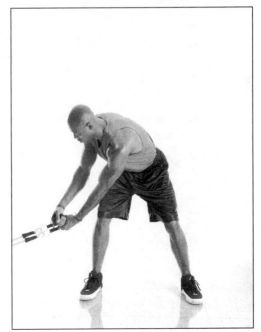

## Exercise 7. Standing Back Rows

**Muscle group targeted:** (Latissimus dorsi)

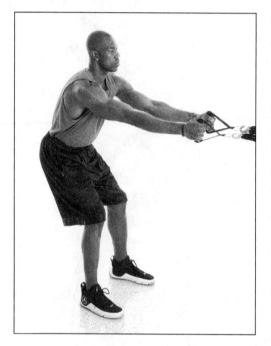

**SETUP/STARTING POSITION:** Anchor a band at waist height. Position your body so that you are facing the anchor point and grip a handle in each hand. Your arms should be straight out in front of you, parallel to the floor. Rotate your hands so that your thumbs are on top. Move far enough away from the anchor point that there is a slight amount of tension on the band. Keep your knees and feet hip-width apart.

**MOVEMENT:**

**Positive Stage:** Keeping your elbows down and your arms tight to your body, pull the handles back to your stomach.

**Negative Stage:** At a controlled speed, return the handles to the starting position.

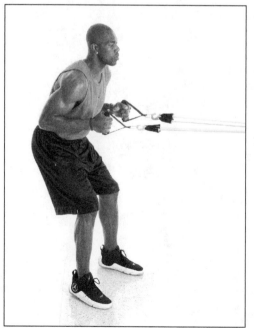

**Buddy's Tip** Another vital muscle group for stronger swings and throws is in the back. Stabilize your center by tightening your stomach muscles and pushing your buttocks forward and upward. To isolate the back muscles, hold the handles with a closed but loose grip.

# GOLF

**FAVORITE GOLFER**: *Hands down, Tiger Woods.*

Many muscles are used in the golf swing. If you strengthen and add power to your chest, arms, stomach, and back, you will be amazed at how much farther the ball will fly. The exercises in this workout are designed to target the muscles required to hit long drives and all other shots in between.

## Program Guidelines

**Frequency:** 3 times per week; for example, Monday, Wednesday, and Friday

**Warm-up and cool-down:** 5 minutes of light cardiovascular work: riding an exercise bike, walking on a treadmill, light jogging, or walking in place

**Sets:** 3 per exercise

**Repetitions (reps) per set:** 18

**Rep speed:** Use a 1 count (say "one-Mississippi" in your head) during the positive stage of the movement and a 2 count (say "one-Mississippi, two-Mississippi" in your head) during the negative stage.

**Breathing:** Be sure to exhale during the positive stage of the movement.

## Making Progress

Keep in mind that you will need to adjust the resistance so that you are struggling on the last rep of your targeted rep number. This will ensure that you get the full benefit from every set.

## Exercise 1. Long-Drive Arm Exercise 1

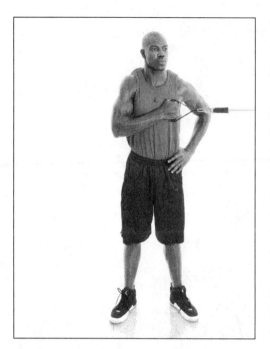

**SETUP/STARTING POSITION:** Anchor a band at chest height. Position your body so that your left shoulder is facing the anchor point and grip the handle (or handles) with your right hand. Your right arm should be across your body so that the handle and the palm of your right hand are just below your left shoulder. Move far enough away from the anchor point that there is a slight amount of tension on the band. Keep your knees slightly bent and your head straight. Place your left hand on your left hip.

**MOVEMENT:**

**Positive Stage:** Pull the handle across your body until your arm is straight out to the side, almost fully extended. Keep your arm raised as you pull so that it is parallel at the end of the pull.

**Negative Stage:** At a controlled speed, bend your arm and return the handle to the starting position.

Complete the desired number of reps and then switch sides.

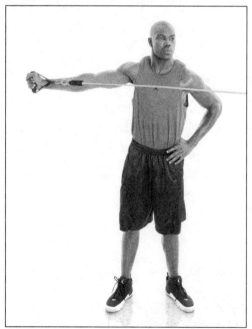

> **Buddy's Tip** Tighten your stomach muscles and push your buttocks forward and upward in your starting position.

## Exercise 2. Long-Drive Chest Exercise 1

**SET UP/STARTING POSITION:** Anchor a band at chest height. Position your body with your back to the anchor point. Grip a handle in each hand and sit on a stability ball. Your palms should be facing down and the band should be above your arms. You should be sitting far enough away from the anchor point that there is a slight amount of tension on the band. Start with your arms parallel with the floor and your elbows bent, creating a 90-degree angle between your forearm and upper arm.

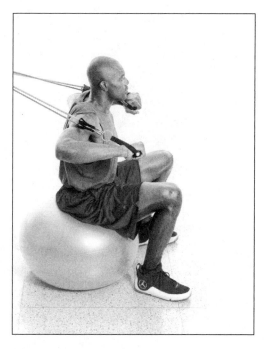

**MOVEMENT:**

**Positive Stage:** Push the handles forward until your arms are almost fully extended.

**Negative Stage:** At a controlled speed, return your arms and the handles to the starting position.

> **Buddy's Tip** When you are sitting on a stability ball, the pelvic tilt will help you remain stable. Tighten your stomach muscles and push your buttocks forward and upward. Try to keep your elbows up and arms parallel with the floor. This will ensure that you work the chest muscles and not the shoulders.

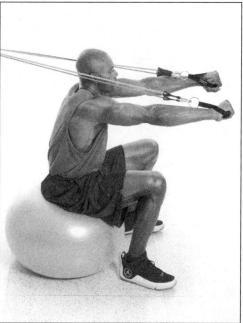

## Exercise 3. Long-Drive Stomach Exercise

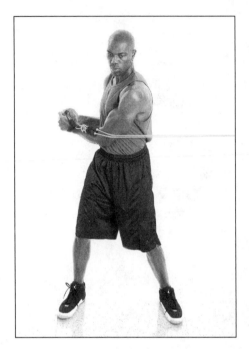

**SETUP/STARTING POSITION:** Anchor a band at stomach height. Grip the handle (or handles) with both hands and turn your body so that your left shoulder faces the anchor point. Move far enough away from the anchor point that there is a slight amount of tension on the band. Hold the handle tight to your stomach just below your ribs. Keep your feet shoulder-width apart and your knees slightly bent.

**MOVEMENT:**

**Positive Stage:** Twist your upper body to the right until it stops naturally.

**Negative Stage:** At a controlled speed, return your upper body to the starting position.

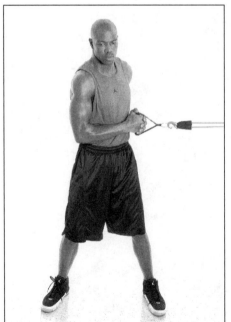

**Buddy's Tip** It is very important to have a strong center as you twist your body. To create the pelvic tilt, tighten your stomach muscles and push your buttock forward and upward. Concentrate on using only your stomach muscles to twist your body; your arms should not do any of the work.

# Exercise 4. Long-Drive Arm Exercise 2

**SETUP/STARTING POSITION:** Stand on a band with your feet hip-width apart. Make sure that the length of the band from the outside of your shoes to the handles is the same on both sides. Grip a handle in each hand and stand up straight. Your arms should be perpendicular to the floor with your palms facing forward. Keep a slight bend in your knees.

**MOVEMENT:**

**Positive Stage:** Keeping your elbows stationary at your sides, raise the handles until they are at chest height.

**Negative Stage:** At a controlled speed, lower the handles to the starting position.

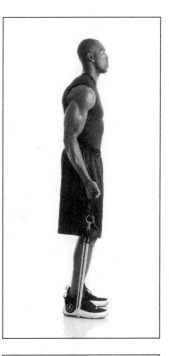

---

**Buddy's Tip** For you to properly isolate and work your biceps, your body must stay still; do not rock your body to raise the handles. One way to help stabilize your body is with—you guessed it—the pelvic tilt: tighten your stomach muscles and push your buttocks forward and upward. Your elbows must stay in one place. Do not move your elbows forward or backward as you raise the handles.

---

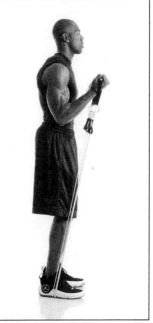

## Exercise 5. Long-Drive Chest Exercise 2

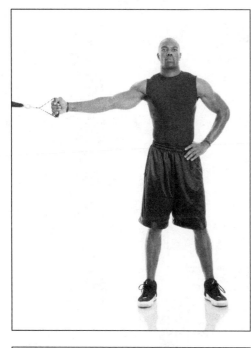

**SETUP/STARTING POSITION:** Anchor a band at chest height and attach both ends to one handle (you can also hold two handles in one hand). Grip the handle with your right hand and turn your body so that your right shoulder is facing the anchor point. Position your right arm out to the side so that it is parallel with the floor and slightly bent. Rotate your wrist so that your thumb is on top. Move your body far enough from the anchor point that there is a slight amount of tension on the band. Keep your left hand on your left hip and your knees slightly bent.

**MOVEMENT:**

**Positive Stage:** Pull the handle out and across your body until it is just past the center of your chest.

**Negative Stage:** At a controlled speed, return the handle to the starting position.

Perform the desired number of reps and then switch sides.

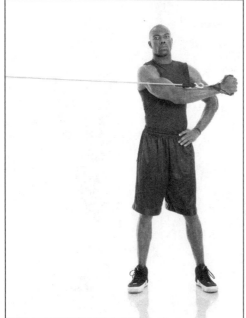

**Buddy's Tip** Tighten your stomach muscles and push your buttocks forward and upward. Do not bend your working arm too much as you pull the handle across your body. Try to imagine that your arm naturally has a slight bend and is fused that way. If you still have trouble, try lowering the amount of resistance.

## Exercise 6. Long-Drive Back Exercise

**Muscle group targeted:** Latissimus dorsi

**SETUP/STARTING POSITION:** Anchor a band at waist height. Position your body so that you are facing the anchor point and grip a handle in each hand. Your arms should be straight out in front of you, parallel with the floor. Rotate your hands so that your thumbs are on top. Move far enough away from the anchor point that there is a slight amount of tension on the band. Keep your knees and feet hip-width apart.

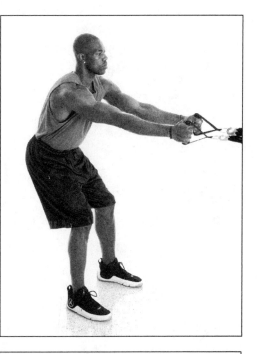

**MOVEMENT:**

**Positive Stage:** Keeping your elbows down and your arms tight to your body, pull the handles back to your stomach.

**Negative Stage:** At a controlled speed, return the handles to the starting position.

> **Buddy's Tip** Create the pelvic tilt by tightening your stomach muscles and pushing your buttocks forward and upward. To isolate your back muscles, hold the handles with a closed but loose grip.

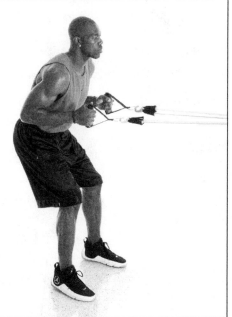

# MARTIAL ARTS

**FAVORITE MARTIAL ARTS ATHLETE:** *I only really know actors.*
*Bruce Lee is still the coldest dude in the game.*

If you practice any of the martial arts, this routine will help you gain the edge over your competition. If you can punch harder, kick harder, and keep your hands up longer to protect yourself, you have a better chance of surviving your fight. The exercises in this routine strengthen the muscles needed for punching, kicking, and blocking. Train your body hard and win!

## Program Guidelines

**Frequency:** 3 times per week; for example, Monday, Wednesday, and Friday

**Warm-up and cool-down:** 5 minutes of light cardiovascular work: riding an exercise bike, walking on a treadmill, light jogging, or walking in place

**Sets:** 3 per exercise

**Repetitions (reps) per set:** Perform 5 to 8 repetitions with a lot of resistance. Then lower the resistance and complete an additional 25 repetitions or keep going until muscle failure.

**Rep speed:** Use a 1 count (say "one-Mississippi" in your head) during the positive stage of the movement and again during the negative stage.

**Breathing:** Be sure to exhale during the positive stage of the movement.

## Making Progress

Keep in mind that you will need to adjust the resistance so that you are struggling on the last rep of your targeted rep number. This will ensure that you get the full benefit from every set.

# Exercise 1. One-Leg Resisted High Kick

**SETUP/STARTING POSITION:** Anchor a band at floor level. Attach one end to an ankle strap and secure it around your right ankle. Position your body with your back to the anchor point. Keep your left foot forward and your hands tight to your body, right below your chest. Move your body far enough away from the anchor point that there is a slight amount of tension on the band.

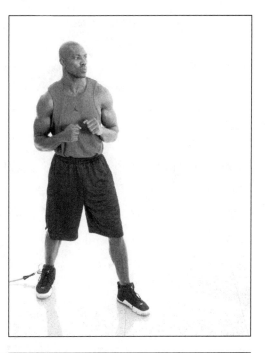

**MOVEMENT:**

**Positive Stage:** Push off from your right leg and kick it forward, up, and to the side until it is almost fully extended.

**Negative Stage:** At a controlled speed, return your right leg to the starting position.

Complete the desired number of reps and then switch sides.

> **Buddy's Tip** This is a very difficult exercise because it requires good balance. However, you can do it! As you are kicking, be sure to pivot your nonkicking foot.

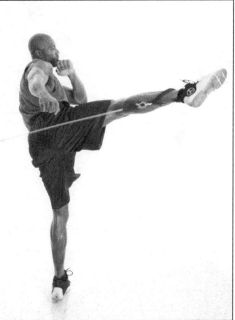

## Exercise 2. Alternating Forward Punch

**SETUP/STARTING POSITION:** Anchor a band at chest height. Position your body with your back to the anchor point. Reach back and grip a handle in each hand. Your hands should be at chest height with your palms facing in toward each other. Keep your upper arms tight to your body and your elbows down. Move your body far enough away from the anchor point that there is a slight amount of tension on the band.

**MOVEMENT:**

**Positive Stage:** Punch forward with your right hand until your arm is almost fully extended and parallel to the floor.

**Negative Stage:** At a controlled speed, return your hand to the starting position.

Switch arms and punch forward with the left hand. Continue to alternate arms until you complete the desired number of reps.

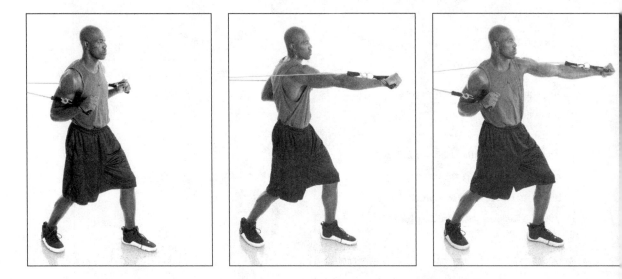

**Buddy's Tip** To properly anchor your lower body, tighten your stomach muscles and push your buttocks forward and upward. As you punch, rotate your hand so that your palm is facing the floor at the end of the movement.

# Exercise 3. Backhand Punch/Block

**SETUP/STARTING POSITION:** Anchor a band at chest height. Position your body so that you are facing the anchor point and grip a handle in each hand. Keep your arms straight out in front of you and parallel with the floor. Rotate your hands so that your thumbs are on top and push your hands together. Your legs should be slightly bent and your head straight. Move your body far enough away from the anchor point that there is a slight amount of tension on the band.

**MOVEMENT:**

**Positive Stage:** Pull the handles out and back until your arms stop naturally.

**Negative Stage:** At a controlled speed, return the handles to the starting position.

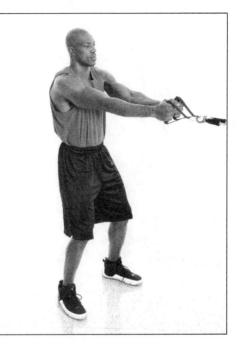

> **Buddy's Tip** To add power to a backhand punch or block, you will need strong rear shoulder muscles. This exercise targets those muscles. To create the pelvic tilt, tighten your stomach muscles and push your buttocks forward and upward.

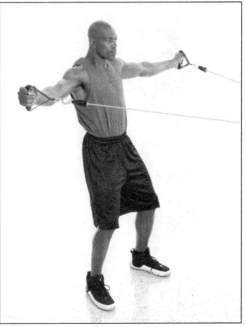

## Exercise 4. Front Block

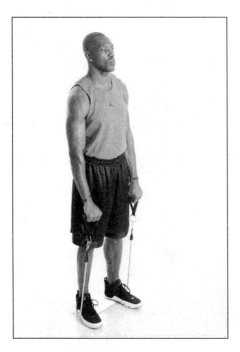

**SETUP/STARTING POSITION:** Stand on a band with your feet hip-width apart. Make sure that the length of the band from the outside of your shoe to the handle is the same on both sides. Grip a handle in each hand and stand up straight with your knees slightly bent. Your arms should be almost fully extended with your hands in front of your thighs. Rotate your wrists so that your palms are facing toward your legs.

**MOVEMENT:**

**Positive Stage:** Raise your arms until they are parallel with the floor.

**Negative Stage:** At a controlled speed, lower your arms to the starting position.

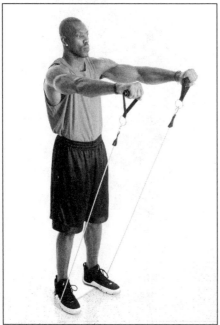

**Buddy's Tip** This exercise is great at strengthening the muscles that are needed to effectively block punches and kicks coming from the front. As you get into your starting position, remember to implement the pelvic tilt: tighten your stomach muscles and pull your buttocks forward and upward. When you raise the handles, try not to bend your arms too much and keep your hands shoulder-width apart.

## Exercise 5. Side Block

**SETUP/STARTING POSITION:**  Stand on a band with your feet hip-width apart. Make sure that the length of the band from the outside of your shoe to the handle is the same on both sides. Reach down and grip a handle in each hand. Stand up straight with your arms at your sides and your palms facing in toward each other. Keep your knees slightly bent.

**MOVEMENT:**

**Positive Stage:**  Raise your arms straight out to the sides until your elbows reach shoulder height.

**Negative Stage:**  At a controlled speed, lower your arms to the starting position.

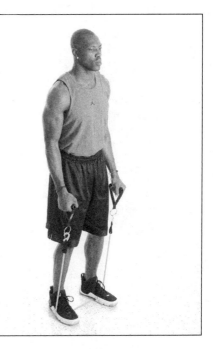

**Buddy's Tip**  This exercise strengthens the muscles that are needed to effectively block punches and kicks coming from the sides. Before you start the movement, create the pelvic tilt by tightening your stomach muscles and pulling your buttocks forward and upward. Keep your elbows higher than your hands as you raise your arms, and imagine that you are pouring milk out of cartons as you raise your arms.

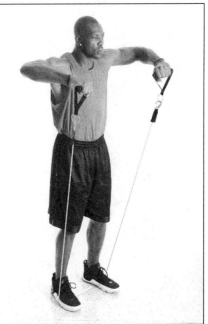

## Exercise 6. Punch Power

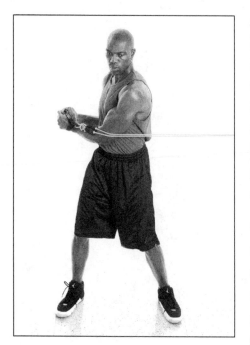

**SETUP/STARTING POSITION:** Anchor a band at stomach height. Grip the handle or handles with both hands and turn your body so that your left shoulder faces the anchor point. Move far enough away from the anchor point that there is a slight amount of tension on the band. Hold the handle tight to your stomach just below your ribs. Keep your feet shoulder-width apart and your knees slightly bent.

**MOVEMENT:**

**Positive Stage:** Twist your upper body to the right until it stops naturally.

**Negative Stage:** At a controlled speed, return your upper body to the starting position.

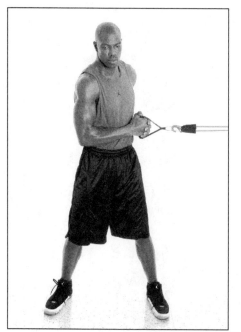

**Buddy's Tip** This exercise is designed to strengthen the core (stomach) muscles that are responsible for adding power and speed to your punches. It is very important to have a strong center as you twist your body. To create the pelvic tilt, tighten your stomach muscles and push your buttocks forward and upward. Concentrate on using only your stomach muscles to twist your body; your arms should not do any of the work.

# TENNIS

**FAVORITE TENNIS PLAYER**: *Gotta give it up to my girls Venus and Serena. Yet, Andy Roddick is the man too.*

To excel at tennis, you need to strengthen and build the muscles that are associated with swinging a racket and moving quickly around the court. Specifically, you will need to condition your shoulders, rotator cuffs, chest, stomach, and legs. The exercises below target all these muscle groups.

## Program Guidelines

**Frequency:** 3 times per week; for example, Monday, Wednesday, and Friday

**Warm-up and cool-down:** 5 minutes of light cardiovascular work; riding an exercise bike, walking on a treadmill, light jogging, or walking in place

**Sets:** 3 per exercise

**Repetitions (reps) per set:** 15

**Rep speed:** Use a 1 count (say "one-Mississippi" in your head) during the positive stage of the movement and again during the negative stage.

**Breathing:** Be sure to exhale during the positive stage of the movement.

## Making Progress

Keep in mind that you will need to adjust the resistance so that you are struggling on the last rep of your targeted rep number. This will ensure that you get the full benefit from every set.

## Exercise 1. Overhead Smash and Serve

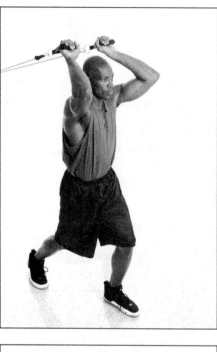

**SETUP/STARTING POSITION:** Anchor a band at chest height. Position your body so that your back is to the anchor point and grip a handle in each hand. Raise your arms so that your elbows are at eye level and shoulder-width apart. Your hands should be above and behind your head with your palms facing forward. Move far enough away from the anchor point that there is a slight amount of tension on the band and put one foot forward.

**MOVEMENT:**

**Positive Stage:** Push the handles forward and up until your arms are almost fully extended.

**Negative Stage:** At a controlled speed, return your arms to the starting position.

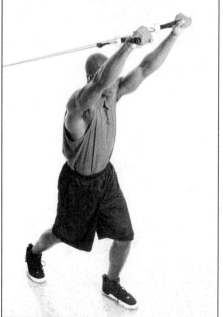

**Buddy's Tip** This exercise improves the strength of the arm muscles, which assist with a downward swing. Create the pelvic tilt by tightening your stomach muscles and pushing your buttocks forward and upward. Keep your hands shoulder-width apart as you push them up and forward.

# Exercise 2. Power Backhand

**SETUP/STARTING POSITION:** Anchor a band at waist height. Position your body so that your chest is facing the anchor point and grip a handle in each hand. Sit on a stability ball. You should be sitting far enough away from the anchor point that there is a slight amount of tension on the band. Keep your arms almost fully extended in front of you and parallel with the floor. Rotate your hands so that your thumbs are on top and push them together. Your knees and feet should be a little more than shoulder-width apart.

**MOVEMENT:**

**Positive Stage:** Keeping your arms parallel with the floor, pull the handles out and back until your arms naturally stop.

**Negative Stage:** At a controlled speed, return the handles to the starting position.

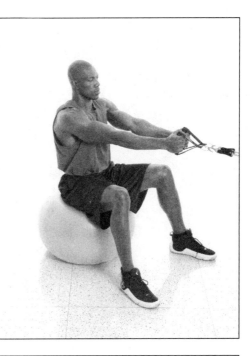

> **Buddy's Tip**  To develop a powerful backhand, you will need to strengthen the back of your shoulders. This exercise targets that specific area. Tighten your stomach muscles and push your buttocks forward and upward. Don't bend your arms as you pull back; try to keep them almost fully extended.

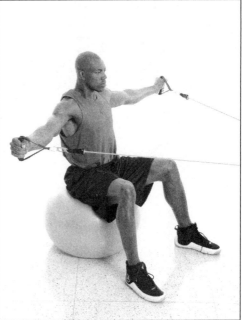

## Exercise 3. Power Forehand

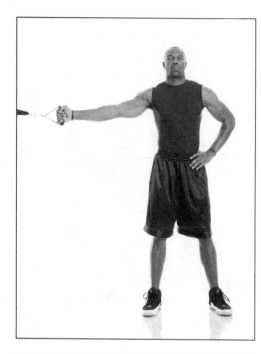

**SETUP/STARTING POSITION:** Anchor a band at chest height and attach both ends to one handle (you could also hold two handles in one hand). Grip the handle with your right hand and turn your body so that your right shoulder is facing the anchor point. Position your right arm out to the side so that it is parallel with the floor with a slight bend. Rotate your hand so that your thumb is on top. Move your body far enough from the anchor point that there is a slight amount of tension on the band. Keep your left hand on your left hip and your knees slightly bent.

**MOVEMENT:**

**Positive Stage:** Pull the handle out and across your body until it is just past the center of your chest.

**Negative Stage:** At a controlled speed, return the handle to the starting position.

Complete the desired number of reps and then switch sides.

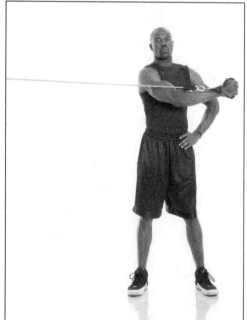

> **Buddy's Tip** A powerful forehand is closely tied to a powerful chest. This exercise effectively works the chest muscles. Tighten your stomach muscles and push your buttocks forward and upward. Do not bend your working arm too much as you pull the handle across your body. Try to imagine that your arm naturally has a slight bend and is fused that way. If you still have trouble, try lowering the amount of resistance.

# Exercise 4. Net Advantage

**SETUP/STARTING POSITION:** Anchor a band at chest height. Position your body so that you are facing the anchor point. Grip the handle with your right hand and raise it to the side so that your arm is parallel with the floor. Your elbow should be bent at a 90-degree angle between your forearm and upper arm. Move your body far enough from the anchor point that there is a slight amount of tension on the band. Position your feet shoulder-width apart and rest your left hand on your left hip.

**MOVEMENT:**

**Positive Stage:** Pull the handle and rotate your arm up until your arm stops naturally.

**Negative Stage:** At a controlled speed, rotate your arm back to the starting position.

Complete the desired number of reps and then switch sides.

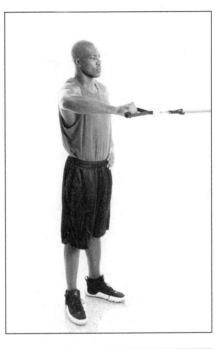

> **Buddy's Tip** When you are at the net, you have to be quick. You will be amazed at how much faster your racket moves after performing this exercise. Create the pelvic tilt by tightening your stomach muscles and pushing your buttocks forward and upward. As you rotate your arm and pull the handle up, try not to move your upper arm forward or backward; keep it straight out to the side.

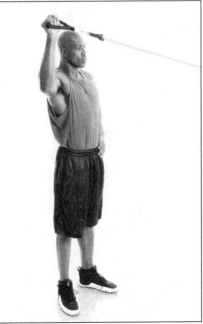

## Exercise 5. Power Serve, Power Smash

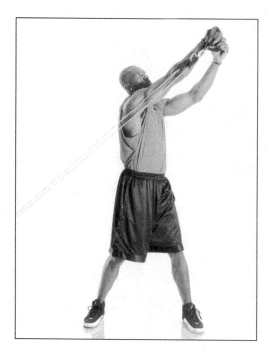

**SETUP/STARTING POSITION:** Anchor a band above your head. Grip the handle (or handles) with both hands and turn your body so that your left shoulder faces the anchor point. Raise the handle up and to the left side so that it is at ear height. Your arms should be up and almost fully extended. Move far enough away from the anchor point that there is a slight amount of tension on the band. Keep your feet shoulder-width apart.

**MOVEMENT:**

**Positive Stage:** Pull the handle down and across your body until it is just past your right knee.

**Negative Stage:** At a controlled speed, return the handle to the starting position.

Complete the desired number of reps and then switch sides.

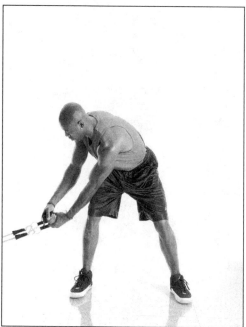

**Buddy's Tip** This exercise will add power to your serve or overhead smash by strengthening the stomach muscles. Remember that this is not an arm exercise. Try to concentrate on using your stomach muscles to pull the handle down and across your body. Your arms should be bent only slightly throughout the exercise.

# Exercise 6. Quick Courtside Shuffle

**SETUP/STARTING POSITION:** Anchor a band at waist height. Position your body so that you are facing the anchor and grip a handle in each hand. Keep your arms out in front of your body with the handles at chest height. Move far enough away from the anchor point that there is a slight amount of tension on the band. Your knees should be shoulder-width apart and slightly bent.

**MOVEMENT:** Shuffle your feet to the right side with small lateral steps until you have traveled 3 to 4 feet. Then shuffle your feet to the left side with small lateral steps, back to the starting position.

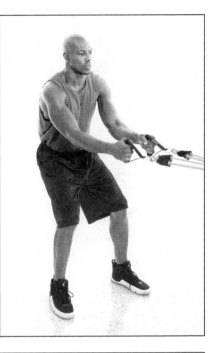

> **Buddy's Tip**  This exercise strengthens the leg muscles. Right before you shuffle, tighten your stomach muscles and push your buttocks forward and upward.

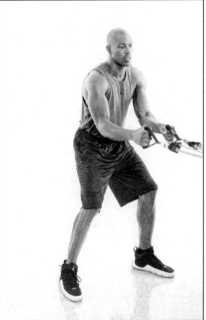

## Exercise 7. Overall Power Swing

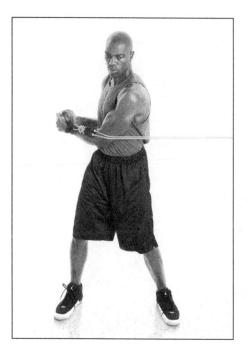

**SETUP/STARTING POSITION:** Anchor a band at stomach height. Grip the handle (or handles) with both hands and turn your body so that your left shoulder faces the anchor point. Move far enough away from the anchor point that there is a slight amount of tension on the band. Hold the handle tight to your stomach just below your ribs. Keep your feet shoulder-width apart and your knees slightly bent.

**MOVEMENT:**

**Positive Stage:** Twist your upper body to the right until it stops naturally.

**Negative Stage:** At a controlled speed, return your upper body to the starting position.

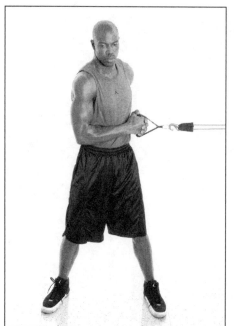

**Buddy's Tip** Whether you need more power in your backhand, your forehand, or both, you will see a big difference with this stomach-strengthening exercise. It is very important to have a strong center as you twist your body. To create the pelvic tilt, tighten your stomach muscles and push your buttocks forward and upward. Concentrate on using only your stomach muscles to twist your body; your arms should not do any of the work.

# BASKETBALL

**FAVORITE BASKETBALL PLAYER**: *The Legendary M. J.*

Basketball, which is my first love as far as sports go, requires great shoulder strength and leg stamina. The players who are able to push past fourth-quarter exhaustion are the ones who dominate. The exercises in this workout target the required muscle groups to help you stay in the game. Within a few weeks you should feel a significant difference on the court.

## Program Guidelines

**Frequency:** 3 times per week; for example, Monday, Wednesday, and Friday

**Warm-up and cool-down:** 5 minutes of light cardiovascular work: riding an exercise bike, walking on a treadmill, light jogging, or walking in place

**Sets:** 3 per exercise

**Repetitions (reps) per set:** 30

**Rep speed:** Use a 1 count (say "one-Mississippi" in your head) during the positive stage of the movement and a 2 count (say "one-Mississippi, two-Mississippi" in your head) during the negative stage.

**Breathing:** Be sure to exhale during the positive stage of the movement.

## Making Progress

Keep in mind that you will need to adjust the resistance so that you are struggling on the last rep of your targeted rep number. This will ensure that you get the full benefit from every set.

## Exercise 1. Resisted Jump

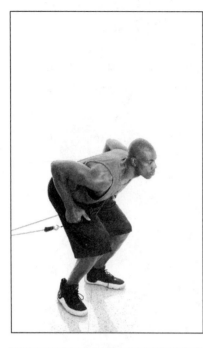

**SETUP/STARTING POSITION:** Anchor a band at floor height. Position your body so that your back is facing the anchor point. Grip a handle in each hand and squat down until your legs are almost parallel with the floor. Keep your arms bent with your palms resting on your thighs. Keep your knees and feet shoulder-width apart. Your chest should be up and your head straight.

**MOVEMENT:**

**Positive Stage:** Jump straight up and then land softly on both feet.

**Negative Stage:** At a controlled speed, squat down to the starting position.

> **Buddy's Tip** It is very easy to let the momentum push you down to a very deep squat on the lowering part of the movement. Try to control the movement, and stop when your thighs are almost parallel with the floor.

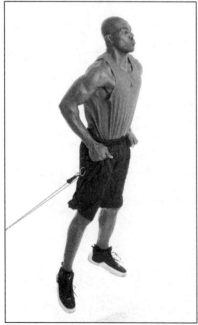

# Exercise 2. Overhead Reach

**SETUP/STARTING POSITION;** Anchor a band at floor level. Grip a handle in each hand and stand up straight. Raise your hands to chest height, shoulder-width apart. Your palms should be facing away from you. Keep your feet and knees shoulder-width apart and your knees slightly bent.

**MOVEMENT:**

**Positive Stage:** Raise your hands straight over your head until your arms stop naturally.

**Negative Stage:** At a controlled speed, lower your hands to the starting position.

> **Buddy's Tips** Tighten your stomach muscles and push your buttocks forward and upward. As you raise your arms, maintain the shoulder-width distance between your hands.

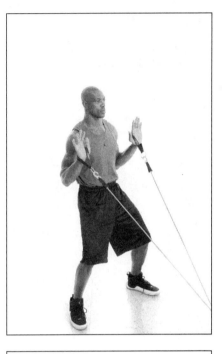

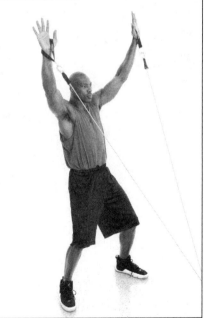

## Exercise 3. Side-to-Side Step-through

**SETUP/STARTING POSITION:**  Anchor a band at knee height. Grip two handles together at chest height. Your elbows should be right by your waist. Move far enough away from the anchor point that there is a slight amount of tension on the band. Keep your knees slightly bent and your head straight.

**MOVEMENT:**

**Positive Stage:**  Take a step back with your right leg while you simultaneously twist your body. End the movement when your hands are behind you and at chest height.

**Negative Stage:**  At a controlled speed, return your hands, body, and right leg to the starting position.

Complete the desired number of reps and then switch sides.

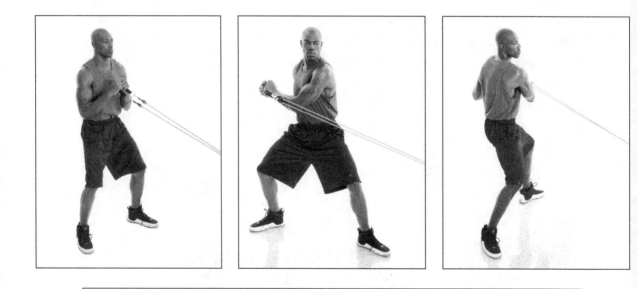

**Buddy's Tip**  Keep your chest up and your head straight as you step back.

## Exercise 4. Forward Two-Arm Push

**SETUP/STARTING POSITION:** Anchor a band at waist height. Position your body so that your back is facing the anchor point. Reach back and grip a handle in each hand. Step forward with one leg. You should be standing far enough away from the anchor point that there is a slight amount of tension on the band. Raise your hands to chest height and rotate them so that your palms are facing down. Keep your hands shoulder-width apart.

**MOVEMENT:**

**Positive Stage:** Push your hands forward until your arms are almost fully extended and parallel with the floor.

**Negative Stage:** At a controlled speed, return your hands to the starting position.

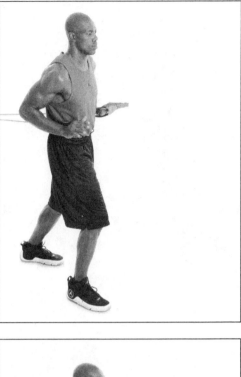

> **Buddy's Tip** Basketball is one of the sports in which you can benefit greatly from a strong center of gravity. Tighten your stomach muscles and push your buttocks forward and upward. Try to imagine that as you are pushing your hands forward, you are making a quick forward pass to a teammate.

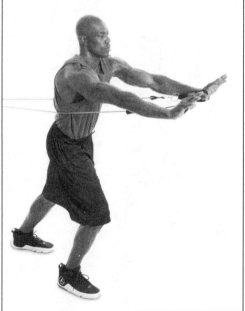

## Exercise 5. Overhead Throw

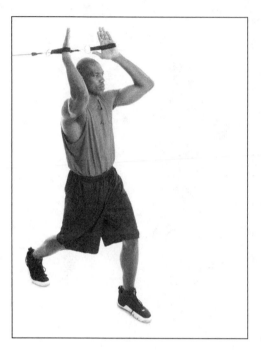

**SETUP/STARTING POSITION:** Anchor a band over your head. Position your body so that your back is facing the anchor point. Reach back and grip a handle in each hand. Place one leg in front and raise your hands over and behind your head. Move far enough away from the anchor point that there is a slight amount of tension on the band. Keep your hands shoulder-width apart and rotate them so that your palms are facing in toward each other.

**MOVEMENT:**

**Positive Stage:** Push your hands up and forward until your arms are almost fully extended and at eye level.

**Negative Stage:** At a controlled speed, return your hands to the starting position.

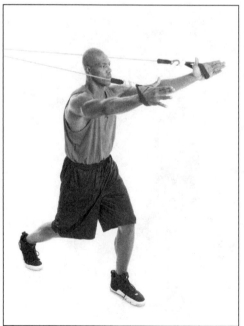

> **Buddy's Tip**  Start by implementing the pelvic tilt: tighten your stomach muscles and push your buttocks forward and upward. As you push, try to keep your hands and elbows shoulder-width apart.

# Exercise 6. Lunge

**SETUP/STARTING POSITION:** Anchor a band at floor level. Face the anchor point and position your legs with your left foot forward. Grip a handle in each hand and raise the handles to shoulder height. Rotate your hands so that your palms are facing forward.

**MOVEMENT:**

**Negative Stage:** At a controlled speed, lower your body straight down until your left thigh is parallel with the floor.

**Positive Stage:** Push from your left heel and raise your body until your left leg is almost straight.

Complete the desired number of reps and switch sides.

> **Buddy's Tip** The knee of your front leg should not move forward during the exercise. To avoid this, concentrate on lowering your hips straight down to the floor.

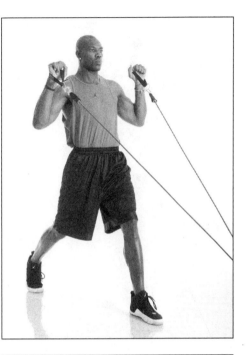

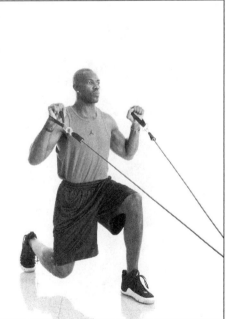

## Exercise 7. Standing Lateral Raise

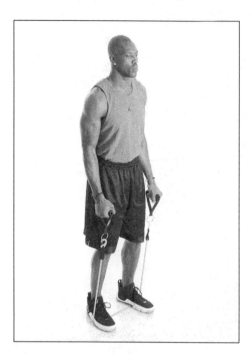

**SETUP/STARTING POSITION:** Stand on a band with your feet hip-width apart. Make sure that the length of the band from the outside of your shoe to the handle is the same on both sides. Reach down and grip a handle in each hand. Stand up straight with your arms at your sides and your palms facing in toward each other. Keep a slight bend in your legs.

**MOVEMENT:**

**Positive Stage:** Raise your arms straight out to the sides until your elbows reach shoulder height.

**Negative Stage:** At a controlled speed, return your arms to the starting position.

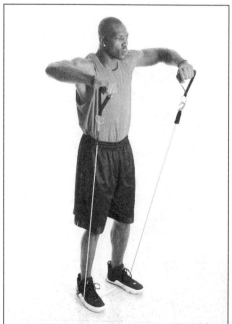

**Buddy's Tip** Before you start the movement, be sure that you create the pelvic tilt by tightening your stomach muscles and pulling your buttocks forward and upward. Keep your elbows higher than your hands as you raise your arms. A great trick to help you use proper form is to imagine that you are pouring milk out of cartons as you raise your arms.

# FOOTBALL

**FAVORITE FOOTBALL PLAYER**: *Jerry Rice will always be at the top of my fab five list. But my list is long 'cause this is what I do!*

Explosive, powerful movements! That's what you need to survive on the football field. The exercises in this workout are designed to help you on the line of scrimmage and beyond.

## PROGRAM GUIDELINES

**Frequency:** 3 times per week; for example, Monday, Wednesday, and Friday

**Warm-up and cool-down:** 5 minutes of light cardiovascular work; riding an exercise bike, walking on a treadmill, light jogging, or walking in place

**Sets:** 3 per exercise

**Repetitions (reps) per set:** 12

**Rep speed:** use a 1 count (say "one-Mississippi" in your head) during the positive stage of the movement and a 2 count (say "one-Mississippi, two-Mississippi" in your head) during the negative stage.

**Breathing:** Be sure to exhale during the positive stage of the movement.

## MAKING PROGRESS

Keep in mind that you will need to adjust the resistance so that you are struggling on the last rep of your targeted rep number. This will ensure that you get the full benefit from every set.

## Exercise 1. Receiver Grab

**SETUP/STARTING POSITION:** Anchor a band at floor level. Position your body so that you are facing the anchor point and grip a handle in each hand. Stand up straight with your knees and feet a little more than shoulder-width apart. Raise your hands to stomach height with your palms facing forward. Keep your hands close together with your thumbs touching and your elbows down at your sides.

**MOVEMENT:**

**Positive Stage:** Push your hands up and to the right side until your arms are almost fully extended.

**Negative Stage:** At a controlled speed, return your hands and arms to the starting position.

Complete the desired number of reps and then switch sides.

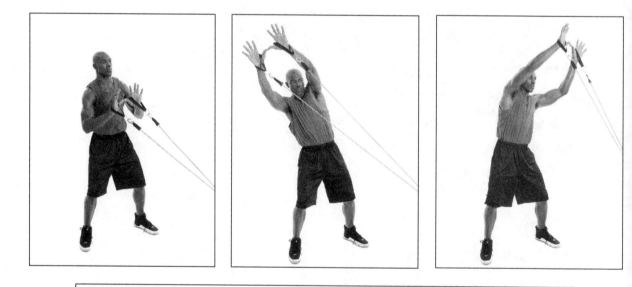

**Buddy's Tip**  This exercise is really great for receivers. Implement the pelvic tilt by tightening your stomach muscles and pushing your buttocks forward and upward.

# Exercise 2. Two-Arm Forward-and-Up Jam

**SETUP/STARTING POSITION:** Anchor a band at knee height. Position your body so that your back is turned to the anchor point and grip a handle in each hand. Stand up straight with one foot forward, keeping a slight bend in your knees. Raise your arms to stomach height and rotate your wrists so that your palms are facing down. Keep your hands shoulder-width apart.

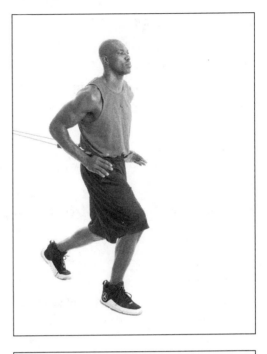

**MOVEMENT:**

**Positive Stage:** Push forward and up until your arms are almost fully extended and your hands are at eye level.

**Negative Stage:** At a controlled speed, return your hands and arms to the starting position.

> **Buddy's Tip** Implement the pelvic tilt by tightening your stomach muscles and pushing your buttocks forward and upward. This exercise is really great for any position that requires you to block or bump an opponent.

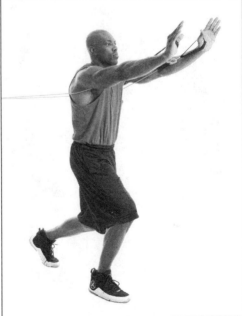

## Exercise 3. Resisted Side Block

**SETUP/STARTING POSITION:**  Anchor a band at floor height. Position your body so that your back is facing the anchor point and grip a handle in each hand. Raise your hands to chest height with your palms facing forward. Keep your arms tight to your body with your elbows down at your sides. Your feet should be a little more than shoulder-width apart, and your knees should be bent slightly.

**MOVEMENT:**

**Positive Stage:**  Step to the right with your right foot and push your hands in the same direction.

**Negative Stage:**  At a controlled speed, return your foot and hands to the starting position.

Complete the desired number of reps and then switch sides.

> **Buddy's Tip**  Keep your hands up and about 12 inches apart as you step to each side. This exercise is great for lateral blocking on the line of scrimmage.

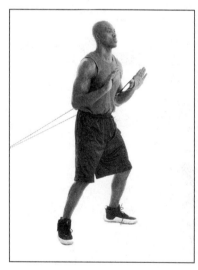 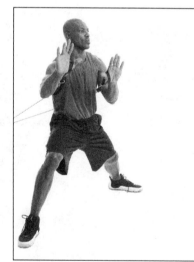 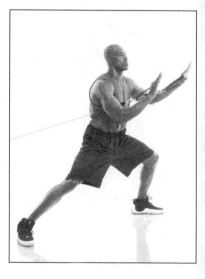

# Exercise 4. Standing One-Arm Chest Fly

**SETUP/STARTING POSITION:** Anchor a band at chest height and attach both ends to one handle (you can also hold two handles in one hand). Grip the handle with your right hand and turn your body so that your right shoulder is facing the anchor point. Position your right arm out to the side so that it is parallel with the floor and slightly bent. Rotate your hand so that your thumb is on top. Move your body far enough from the anchor point that there is a slight amount of tension on the band. Keep your left hand on your left hip and your knees slightly bent.

**MOVEMENT:**

**Positive Stage:** Pull the handle out and across your body until it is just past the center of your chest.

**Negative Stage:** At a controlled speed, return the handle to the starting position.

Complete the desired number of reps and then switch sides.

> **Buddy's Tip** Tighten your stomach muscles and push your buttocks forward and upward. Do not bend your working arm too much as you pull the handle across your body. Try to imagine that your arm naturally has a slight bend and is fused that way. If you still have trouble, try lowering the amount of resistance.

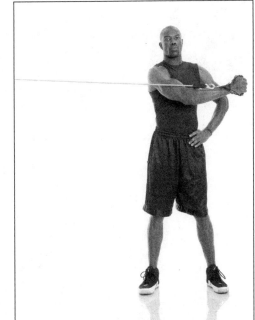

## Exercise 5. Seated Back Row

**Muscle group targeted:** Latissimus dorsi

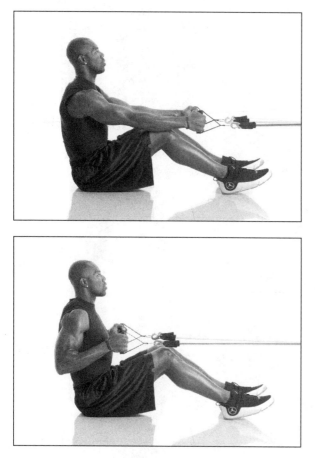

**SETUP/STARTING POSITION:** Anchor a band at knee height. Grip a handle in each hand and face the anchor point. Sit down with your knees bent and your heels on the floor. Move far enough away from the anchor point that there is a slight amount of tension on the band. Your arms should be straight out in front of you, parallel with the floor. Rotate your wrists so that your thumbs are on top.

**MOVEMENT:**

**Positive Stage:** Pull the handles back with your elbows down and your arms tight to your body.

**Negative Stage:** At a controlled speed, return the handles to the starting position.

> **Buddy's Tip**  Do not grip the handles tightly, since this will cause you to start pulling with your biceps instead of your back. Keep your hands closed but loose around the handles.

# Exercise 6. Lunge

**SETUP/STARTING POSITION:** Anchor a band at floor level. Face the anchor point and position your legs with your left foot forward. Grip a handle in each hand and raise the handles to shoulder height. Rotate your hands so that your palms are facing forward.

**MOVEMENT:**

**Negative Stage:** At a controlled speed, lower your body straight down until your left thigh is parallel with the floor.

**Positive Stage:** Push from your left heel and raise your body until your left leg is almost straight.

Complete the desired number of reps and then switch sides.

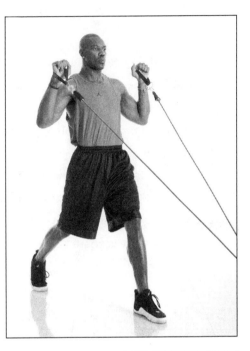

> **Buddy's Tip**  The knee of your front leg should not move forward during the exercise. To avoid this, concentrate on lowering your hips straight down to the floor.

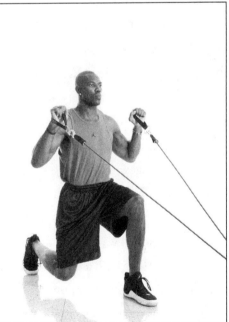

---

**T.O. TESTIMONY:** *Team T.O.*

---

With everything there is a start and a finish. Some people reading this book have followed my career and been a part of my team from the beginning. Others, by reading this book, have just begun their journey to finding fitness.

Below are a few people who shared with us their thoughts, concerns, and fitness goals.

Today marks the beginning of a new journey in this game we call life. Together we're working to become stronger, faster, and better overall. This book is dedicated to those wanting to find fitness. As we take the first step together, the following testimonies share how others define and find fitness for themselves.

---

## YOLANDA TAYLOR, TEAM T.O. WINNER

When asked, "What does fitness mean to me?" I immediately think of my early years when I was a track athlete dedicated to being in the best physical and mental shape possible. Today it means recapturing that dedication with commitment to exercising the mind as well as the body; dedicating time to **both,** just as you do to paying your bills and going to work. It means developing a sensible "life program" that includes working out at least three times a week and planning daily meals that are healthy and work well in conjunction with my metabolism. In addition, fitness means paying attention to my body as it ages and making the right changes in my exercise and eating regimen to compensate for those changes.

My current workout routine consists of an aerobic workout or three miles of walking (treadmill or actual walking) at least three days per week. As a part of the Fitness Ministry at my church, I am with a trainer each Saturday morning for two hours of stretching, stepping, and exercise reps that consist of crunches, leg raises, and push-ups.

My long-term fitness goals are to lose 50 pounds, drop several dress sizes, reduce my body fat, and tone my stomach and thighs. I intend to do this by increasing the intensity of my workouts and incorporating regular visits to the gym for weight training, all while maintaining *at least* a three-day-per-week workout regimen and developing conscientious eating habits.

My future fitness goals are to become so dedicated to my personal fitness program that it becomes second nature and a normal part of my life. I would also like to be an inspiration to friends and associates who are struggling with achieving and maintaining physical and mental fitness.

## JOHN HEART, 43, CEO/ FOUNDER OF TRAINING WITH HEART

Fitness to me is a condition in which good health is maintained as well as a high level of muscular strength, endurance, flexibility, and the ability to perform and recover from any chosen activity in the course of any given day.

My own workout is cyclical in nature. Over the course of six-to-eight-week cycles, I train very intensely with weights. The actual number of workout days is low, but it is necessary for full recovery from the workouts I do. Being a drug-free bodybuilder, I generate a decent amount of intensity, which requires those rest days.

My long-term goal is to be healthy and prosperous and look like it as well. I'd also like to continue to be an example for my clients as well as others around me and encourage them to go for their own dreams and desires with God leading their way!

## RODRICK, 40ISH, CELEBRITY/ CORPORATE PUBLIC RELATIONS

I'm a fortysomething ex–Army sergeant who has stayed in top shape all my life. I realized early that pumping iron would eventually take a toll on my body, and my greatest fear became true when I injured my shoulder.

Instead of spending excessive amounts of money on treatment, I invested in Bodylastics' Terrell Owens Super Strong Man Edition, and I will never be the same. It has helped me to concentrate on specific muscle groups with ease and has helped in my rehabilitation. I'm in the best shape of my life—stronger, faster, injury-free—and I have money in the bank!

## CHRISTOPHER DA SILVA, 42, PRESIDENT AND CEO, NEEDABLANK.COM

Fitness means being able to keep up with my son and staying on top of my health. Being a diabetic for fifteen years makes me appreciate the time I have here now and in the future. The more I exercise, the more I realize how beneficial it is to my long-term health. Finding new ways to break the monotony of having to exercise is always challenging, which is why I welcome and appreciate this book.

My long-terms goals are to break my dependency on insulin and replace it with exercise. In the future, I hope to be a voice to others who don't like to exercise or just don't do so, to help them see the importance of staying in shape and living a long life.

## MAME TWUMASI, 30-SOMETHING, VISUAL MERCHANDISING MANAGER, NIKE

I'm not sure what to say about working out—my intense athlete training days are long over, and I can't say I am very consistent right now. However, this book inspires me to know that I can start where I am and work myself back to where I want to be.

My posttrack days at UCLA allowed my mind and body to quickly embrace even the most challenging of workouts of today, simply because when I do work out, I'm used to working out long and hard. Completing several intense workouts made me physically and mentally tough. Now when any physical pain or turmoil arises, I often tell myself that this is nothing compared to basic training!

From that time, I discovered the best workout for me is the bike. Interval training on the bike used to be one of the most grueling of the lethal workouts. Full speed for twenty to sixty minutes every day for two-plus weeks will shed pounds like nobody's business. I plan to use this strategy when I am blessed with the need to shed postbirth pounds!

For me, a more cardio-driven workout is my exercise of choice. I'm at my best when I am on a team, so I welcome the task of finding fitness, as a new addition to Team T.O.

## CAMILLE CANNON, 37, SURGICAL PHYSICIAN ASSISTANT, WIFE, AND NEW MOTHER

Fitness to me means exercising, eating healthy, and relaxing by meditation, prayer, or sleep. My fitness routine is not as consistent as it needs to be; I am a new mother of an eight-month-old son.

I enjoy the concept of finding fitness and applaud Mr. Owens for taking such a huge step to speak out to individuals who aren't in elite shape. I'm learning that all the things I like to do can be what make up my fitness routine.

Having studied medicine in the military, I'm no stranger to rigorous training, both mentally and physically, which has turned me off to traditional forms of exercises. My favorite exercise is dancing with a class. This could be aerobic dance, salsa dance, ballet, or other kinds of dance.

My fitness goals are to become more consistent in my routine of working out, eating healthfully and getting the proper rest/relaxation time. I would like to see myself at a fitness level where I can run for thirty minutes without stopping. Since both my husband and I decided to have kids a bit later than originally planned, it's important to me to be able to keep up with the physical requirements of parenting a toddler. The way I see it, I will have to start now, because every day, my son is getting closer and closer to two!

## LEONIA COLLINS, 58, ASSISTANT STANFORD MANAGEMENT GROUP, MOTHER OF THREE, GRANDMOTHER OF TWO

Fitness to me is living long, being lean and strong. These are things that I wish to acquire as I get older. I want to be a sexy and healthy grandmother who is able to enjoy and spend quality time with my grandchildren.

I like the concept of finding a fitness routine that works for me and not feeling as though I have to compete with twenty- or thirty-something women who haven't lived to be almost sixty years old.

I know that I can do anything I put my mind to, yet I enjoy a workout that's more relaxing and fun.

Currently, I like to participate in activities like swimming, dancing, and running around with the grandkids.

I try to walk 1.5 miles a day, sometimes 2 miles, three or four times a week. I also do a twelve-minute core workout three times a week, yet I'm not as consistent as I'd like to be. Although I do enjoy working out independently, my preference is to work out with a group of my peers. I'm hoping that this book will inspire my friends to participate in taking the T. O. Challenge together.

## ANGELA BROWN, 31,
## PERSONAL TRAINER, TAILORED-FITNESS,
## MOTHER OF TWO DAUGHTERS, AGES 4 AND 1

Fitness to me is a lifestyle. That is what I teach and have taught for years. It's the one good habit that keeps you healthy and strong.

Usually when people take on a fitness endeavor, they are looking for a simple result: to look good! Yet that can't be the only aspect to fitness, which is what T. O. teaches us through this book.

Fitness incorporated into a lifestyle can bring about a bond with family, friends, and self. Fitness can give you personal accomplishments that no one can take away from you.

I encourage people to look their best self by tapping into their own potential.

As far as my own personal workout, after having had a baby less then a year ago, I've decreased my workout from an hour to a half hour. I try to use Mother Nature as my source of strength, getting outside and embracing nature with a brisk walk or nice jog.

My long-term goals are to influence as many people as possible to invest in themselves (mind, body, and spirit) now versus later. I would like to encourage people to make more conscious choices for their lifestyle and fewer excuses. This goal is not only for them but for me as well. Thanks, T. O., for allowing me the opportunity not only to grow up in knowledge but also to show up in good health.

_____

# Cool-down

**Before we cool down,** keep in mind that the cool-down is designed to bring the mind, body, and spirit together to celebrate your overall accomplishments. Take a deep breath. Relax! Allow your mind, body, and spirit to be free. You did it!

---

**Buddy's Tip** It is important to cool down at the end of any exercise routine. A cool-down is an activity or movement that brings your heart rate down gradually. Why is this so important? Because when you exercise, your heart rate increases. If you simply stop moving abruptly, your heart rate drops very quickly. This can be a shock to your system. However, if you bring your heart rate down gradually, your body has time to adjust. A great way to cool down is simply to walk at a comfortable pace for two minutes.

After you're done walking, you will want to move into the next stage of the cool-down: light stretching.

There are many reasons I feel it is important to stretch at the end of your workout. First, stretching promotes better blood flow to the muscles. During your workout, you place your muscles under new stresses. Increasing blood flow can help with healing and recovery.

Second, stretching helps to counteract the constant forces that pull at the body. Gravity compresses your joints throughout the day. Stretching helps put the body in traction and temporarily take some pressure off the joints.

Last, I have found through experience that stretching after exercise will result in more peace of mind and homeostasis.

---

**Guidelines:** Perform each stretch for 1 minute and then move on to the next one.

**Breathing:** Make sure to breathe comfortably and naturally.

## Exercise 1. Yoga Cat Stretch

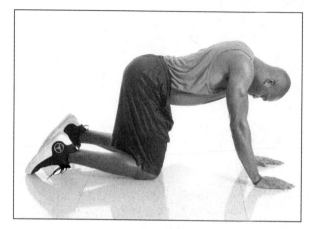

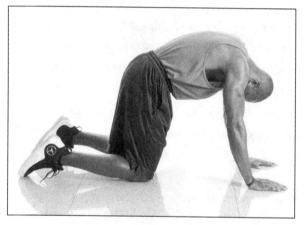

**SETUP/STARTING POSITION:** Kneel on all fours. Keep your elbows in line with your shoulders and your knees under your hips. Your back should be as flat as possible with a slight downward arch.

**STRETCH:** Exhale and push your stomach out as far as it will go. Then inhale and pull your navel in, rounding your back up toward the ceiling like an angry cat, drawing your chin toward your navel.

# Exercise 2. Lotus Position

**SETUP/STARTING POSITION:** Sit on the floor with your back against the wall. Keep your feet together and pulled in toward your groin. Your knees should be up, and your hands should be relaxed at your sides with your knuckles on the floor.

**STRETCH:** Let gravity pull your knees down naturally.

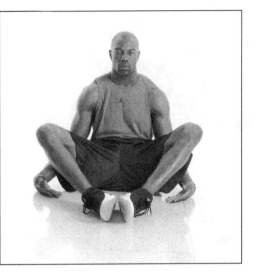

> **Buddy's Tip** Do not bounce your legs, push your legs down, or lean forward. I want you to stretch passively. If you are in the right position, gravity will do the work for you. Breathe normally and naturally.

## Exercise 3. Seated Down-the-Middle Stretch

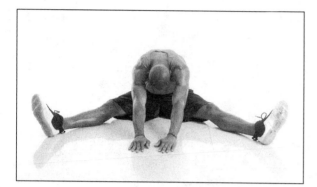

**SETUP/STARTING POSITION:** Sit on the floor with your legs spread wide and your toes pointing up. Keep your arms shoulder-width apart and straight out in front of you. Your palms should be flat on the floor and close to your groin.

**STRETCH:** Pull your upper body forward, moving your hands away from your body.

**Buddy's Tip** Do not bounce forward. To move your upper body forward, lean gently or simply let gravity pull you down. Breathe normally and naturally.

## Exercise 4. Hanging Stretch

**SETUP/STARTING POSITION:** Grip a pole (or any place you can hold your hands above your head) and hold on with both hands. Your arms should be 1 to 2 inches more than shoulder-width apart. Keep your head straight.

**STRETCH:** Hang straight down to the floor.

> **Buddy's Tip**  You can place your feet on the floor as you perform this stretch. Keep a closed but loose grip on the bar and try to relax all of your muscle groups. Elongate your body.

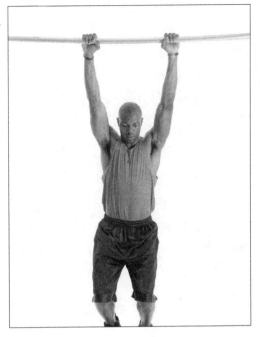

# Fourth Quarter

**It's the fourth quarter,** and there are exactly two minutes left in the game. As we prepare to celebrate another victory, it's important that we reflect on all the hard work that got us to this level.

I want each and every one of you to know that fitness starts with the mind, and mentally, if you've made it to the end of this book, you've already taken the first step toward victory. I am confident that each step forward will bring you closer to your ultimate goal. Good job!

You are a winner! Congratulations!

# Index